pulse

voices from the heart of medicine

more voices
—a second anthology

9/29/12

To Jim—

A FELLOW WRITER,

WARMLY,

Paul Cross

Voices from the Heart of Medicine, Inc.
28 Albert Place
New Rochelle, NY 10801
USA

www.pulsemagazine.org

ISBN - 13: 978-1479309603

Cover and interior design and production by
Laurie Douglas Graphic Design (www.lauriedouglas.com)

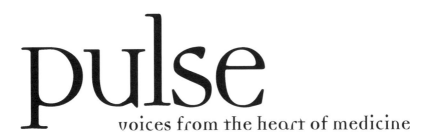

pulse
voices from the heart of medicine

more voices
—a second anthology

Paul Gross MD and Diane Guernsey

Foreword by Maureen Bisognano
President and CEO, Institute for Healthcare Improvement

Introductions by Johanna Shapiro PhD and
Judy Schaefer RNC MA

contents

Fall

Winter

Spring

Summer

Fall

Winter

Indexes

acknowledgments

Pulse is a group effort. The weekly publication and this book have enjoyed the contributions of many people—writers who send us terrific stories and poems, advisors who offer wise counsel and come up with spot-on book titles, friends who tell us how vital *Pulse* is to them, and supporters who introduce *Pulse* to new audiences and whose generosity keeps *Pulse* thriving.

Here are just a few of the many who deserve recognition. We would like to thank...

Two institutions, Montefiore Medical Center and Albert Einstein College of Medicine, whose leadership fosters the kind of creative and humanistic impulses that have allowed *Pulse* to take root and to flourish.

Marti Grayson, Senior Associate Dean for Medical Education at Albert Einstein College of Medicine, for her wisdom, encouragement and support.

Beth Hadas, for her deft and capable editing.

Deby Finkelstein, who joined *Pulse* as an intern just as we were in the final stages of assembling this collection and whose invaluable contributions helped carry *More Voices* to completion.

Larry Bauer and Alice Fornari, the newest members of Voices from the Heart of Medicine, Inc.'s Board of Directors, for their energetic and unshakable belief in *Pulse*.

Every member of the *Pulse* Advisory Group, for offering useful counsel and for (once more) coming up with the perfect title for a *Pulse* anthology.

The *Pulse* writers, whose honesty, courage and creative talent make *Pulse* what it is.

Maureen Bisognano, President and CEO of the Institute for Healthcare Improvement, for literally bringing *Pulse* to work with her—and for letting people know she does that.

Johanna Shapiro and Judy Schaefer, *Pulse*'s poetry editors, for their sensitivity and sensibility, which make them such a joy to collaborate with.

Laurie Douglas for her dazzling and inspired book design and for her unfailing wit, wisdom and patience.

Stephen Yorke, whose web design is the engine that enables *Pulse* to reach so many readers and whose thoughtfulness, humor and creativity make him a pleasure to work with.

And finally, we once again thank Peter Selwyn, Chair of the Department of Family and Social Medicine at Montefiore Medical Center and Albert Einstein College of Medicine. His vision of health care as an agent of humanity, self-awareness and social change has inspired *Pulse*, while his support and friendship have made *Pulse* possible.

to our parents,

Helen and Ros Guernsey, Titine and Joseph Gross,

our very first healers

foreword

Everyone has stories to tell. Here is one of mine.

When my brother Johnny was seventeen years old, he was diagnosed with Hodgkin's disease. It progressed quickly, and he was in and out of hospitals regularly over the next several years.

When Johnny was twenty, he came to my apartment (I was twenty-three) and told me, "I'm not gonna make it."

He was ready to face death, but I wasn't. I didn't know what to say or do. All I could think of doing was to offer encouragement and try to give him hope.

But Johnny stopped me.

"Can I tell you what I want?" he said.

"What do you want?" I asked him.

"I want to turn twenty-one," he said.

Johnny did turn twenty-one, and he died just a few days after that birthday.

Throughout that last year of his life, I still didn't grasp the power of that simple question that Johnny wanted me to ask: "What do you want?"

Looking back, I wonder what might have come from asking that question sooner. I wonder about the people Johnny would've wanted to meet and see. I wonder about the conversations they might have had. And I wonder about the functionality he could have had, to the extent he could, if he'd been able to stay out of the hospital.

Instead of getting his wishes that last year, doing the things he'd wanted to do, and living the way he would have wished, Johnny spent it mostly in the hospital.

I finally saw that question acted on—by a radiation oncologist. When Johnny was in the hospital during that last year of his life, doctors would come and go into and out of his room. They'd speak over him, and about him, but almost never *to* him.

Finally, this radiation oncologist came into my brother's room and asked him, "Johnny—what do you want?"

"I want to go home," Johnny answered.

The doctor then took my leather jacket from me, put it on Johnny, picked him up from his hospital bed and carried him to my car.

Johnny came home, and he spent his final days surrounded by the friends and family who loved him.

That one interaction between Johnny and the radiation oncologist taught me not to rely on just providing encouragement and hope. These things are important, but more important, almost always, is having the conversation with our loved ones about what they want.

That conversation needs to happen more often—within families and between patients and health professionals.

As a former nurse, I know some of the obstacles that get in the way of this conversation.

In the hectic world of medicine, it's easy, almost natural to become absorbed in tasks. Moving from this procedure to that exam to yet another blood-test analysis...the pace is overwhelming. And health care is at once physically taxing, intellectually demanding and emotionally draining. It's easy to lose sight of the prize. It's hard to keep your head, your heart and your hands connected, so that you can care deeply and well for those in need.

This book speaks to me as a former nurse, as someone now devoted to improving health care and as someone who lost a brother at a young age.

What you'll read in this amazing book are personal stories of discovering our vulnerabilities and becoming more effective caregivers. You'll read about clinicians who pause that extra moment and take a hand off the doorknob in order to learn (or teach) a bit more. You'll read about illness and how patients find comfort (or not) from the care they receive. You'll read about loss and about the ways that we heal.

If you are a health professional, this book may change you; it may reconnect you with your professional passion. If you're not a health professional but, like all of us, have friends and family, you'll find yourself in these pages, supporting or needing support, asking or guiding, looking within or reaching out. And if you're a patient, caregiver or simply someone who loves good stories, the book may inspire you to slow down, to take stock, to reconnect with yourself and your loved ones--in short, to feel the pulse of medicine.

Enjoy!

Maureen Bisognano
President and CEO
Institute for Healthcare Improvement (IHI)

introductions

Pulse—voices from the heart of medicine is a unique e-magazine that sends subscribers (for free!) brief weekly readings of original, medically themed prose or poetry. *Pulse* is the inspiration of Paul Gross. Its realization has required the editorial gifts of his wife, Diane Guernsey, and the involvement of a truly impressive group of professionals and laypersons.

Many of you reading this already know the feelings of anticipation that stir as you await *Pulse*'s arrival in your inbox—the sense of curiosity about that week's piece, and the pleasure of savoring it once it arrives. The selection may be inspiring, heartrending or both. But it is always a joy, because it draws you inexorably closer to the heart—even the soul—of medicine.

Pulse has a distinctive orientation. First, it has a very specific focus: It is devoted to writing about experiences of giving and receiving health care. Second, it seeks out many voices—those of patients, nurses, doctors, family members and other caregivers—and makes no distinction between these different groups on the basis of status or hierarchy. Third, *Pulse* stresses authenticity: It wants its authors to truly "speak from the heart," to reflect on deeply felt personal experience in a way that is "true" and "real." Fourth, because medicine has to do (at least theoretically) with healing, *Pulse* aims to be a healing presence in the world of health care, which is so abundant in suffering, for both patients and those who care for them.

Contributors to *Pulse* share their journeys through health or illness, or at least slivers of these journeys, in memorable images and situations that linger in the mind's eye because they are about something much greater than the moment described.

This kind of narrative healing benefits readers and writers in every category—the patients distressed by their bodies' betrayals (and at times, sadly, by the betrayals of the healthcare system itself), and the doctors, nurses and other health professionals who, in caring for these patients under often frustrating and constraining circumstances, can end up feeling burned-out and disillusioned. For all involved, we hope that *Pulse* will be felt as a gift—a small, humanizing act of generosity in a world seemingly preoccupied with billing and insurance coverage, fees and charges.

As one of *Pulse*'s two poetry editors, I've had my own journey with the magazine, having been on board since its inception. (In fact, Paul invited me on board before we knew where the boat was going, or even what kind of boat it was!)

Together with Paul, Diane and my invaluable co-editor, Judy Schaefer, I've had the privilege of working to realize *Pulse*'s vision—and even, at times, helping to shape it.

We are an eclectic (some might say ragtag) band. To use the current phrase, we are "interprofessional." Paul is a family physician, writer and singer-songwriter. Diane is a writer, editor, psychoanalyst and classically trained pianist. Judy is an acclaimed nurse-poet. I am a psychologist by training, one with a great interest in the role of literature in medicine. (I also scribble the occasional poem when I think no one is looking.)

Our freewheeling interdisciplinary exchanges are one of the things I like most about *Pulse*. We are not bound by a single academic worldview; rather, we bring a range of perspectives, likes and dislikes to the process of selecting *Pulse*'s pieces. Although we each contribute a different expertise to the task, we share an essentially democratic attitude toward literature: We believe that stories and poetry are written primarily for ordinary people, and not for literary critics. Despite our regard for "craft" and "wordsmithing" (two words I've learned to value as a result of my interactions with my colleague Judy), we recognize that a compelling story or poem must also offer something more profound: a deeper truth that emanates from the core of the writer's being.

This commitment to seeking out deeper truths sparks the kind of provocative dialogue that occurs with some regularity at *Pulse* and that I find very exciting to take part in: What, really, do we mean by "truth"?

Philosophers have grappled with that question, and so has the staff at *Pulse*. "What is truer than the truth?" asks an old folk saying—and the answer is, "A good story."

But how do we know a story is "true"? At *Pulse*, we ask contributors to confirm that their stories, whether prose or poetry, are based on actual experience. But once the forces of storytelling, craft and wordsmithing take over, a good narrative can never be purely literal. It is shaped by the demands of aesthetics and authorial intent, and by something both more powerful and less under conscious control than either of these—the creator's compelling need to speak or discover his or her own, uniquely personal version of the experiences he's describing. When reading *Pulse*'s many wonderful submissions, we look for the presence of something "truer than truth"—a presence that humbles us when we find it.

Reflecting on our many exchanges (ultimately unresolvable, but rich and fruitful) about the nature of truth leads me inevitably to *Pulse*'s poetry.

As William Carlos Williams famously wrote, "You cannot get the news from poetry." If that's the case, then why read it? Especially in medicine, with its randomized, double-blind, controlled trials and its smartphone apps to aid in clinical decision-making, what good, really, is poetry? Poetry seems uncomfortably non-utilitarian, lacking in measurable outcomes.

Poetry, like prose, is about healing. And everyone involved in health care is in need of healing—patients, families, doctors and nurses alike. I discovered this for myself during various personal encounters with illness, when the research literature I consulted informed but did not console me. Only the bright, sharp edge of Jane Kenyon's verse or the pure uncompromising voice of Raymond Carver could do that. Or lines like these, from one of the poems in this collection, Jan Jahner's "Semi-Private Room," about a nurse's encounter with an anorexic young patient:

> Sometimes nectar appears
> when stories intersect:
> ......

> Our connection becomes a spoon
> with its delicate curve
> Starting the goodbyes, I hand her my card

> she reads through the menu
> departing, I feel the full moon
> rising in my chest.

Prose can do much the same thing, of course, but for me, at least, poetry is a kind compressed truth—"Truth at a slant," as Emily Dickinson put it.

Much of the last fifteen years of my career has been devoted to reading and reflecting on poetry written by patients, medical students and physicians, and talking to some of these poets about why they write. One thing I've learned from this immersion is that poetry is full of surprises, not least for its authors.

Listen to how Stanley Schuman, a pediatrician, is surprised by a puff of grace in this excerpt from his poem "The Ancients Had It Right":

> Consider my distress, in my just-opened pediatric office.
> Stumped by Angela, a three-year-old
> So panicked by my white coat, no way to examine her.
>
> Screaming, clutching Mother, she knew and I knew
> This wasn't university-hospital, with back-up nurses.
> Instead, it was one-on-one,
> Advantage Angela.
>
> Desperate, I felt for a stray balloon in my
> Pants pocket (from my own child's birthday).
> Putting it to my lips, I strained to inflate the stubborn thing.
> Instantly, Angela's tear-reddened eyes opened wide.
> The more I flushed and puffed, clown-like,
> The more she giggled, finally bursting into laughter,
> Sans fear, forgetting pain.
> My breath, a yellow balloon, a child's laughter...
> Three gifts from the gods!

Poetry is often more unexpected, less conventional than prose. It feeds on metaphor, image and sound. Also, good poetry is uncomfortable to read and to create; it is indirect, allusive, ambiguous and open to multiple (sometimes conflicting) interpretations. As I like to remind poetry-resistant learners, poems are a lot like some patients. We might wish that patients resembled a tightly structured, well-developed essay, but often they are more like a poem—hard to grasp, providing only tantalizing hints of themselves, with great complexity packed into a brief space.

In this excerpt from the poem "Dissolution," author Jocelyn Jiao attributes her own metaphoric corrosion of language as a sympathetic resonance to a loved one's dying struggle to speak. "Even fish can sing," the poet writes. As we ponder possible (and impossible) meanings of this elliptical, poignant phrase, we realize how mysterious yet essential the process is by which words connect us.

> it all started at your
> bedside, when your lips
> were parted, straining
> to form one first, final word.
> a sudden embrace of cold
> concrete made you into
> some bright thing with eyes
> translucent, gasping
> for the comfort of
> water, empty and clear—
> when ebullience
> once spilled from your lips
> as a sun warms an earth.
>
> do you see? words are meant
> for creatures of air. i have no use for them;
> even fish can sing.

It is the opportunity to disseminate poetry that wrestles with life and death, suffering and joy, relational detachment and connection, all within the context of medicine, that keeps me ardent about *Pulse*.

Admittedly, it can be terribly difficult to choose from among poems devoted to these grand themes (my co-editor Judy has set the bar very high for "death" poems, since, in her view, the subject gives the writer an unfair advantage over those who have tackled more prosaic topics!). But I love the idea that anyone—doctor, patient, nurse, caregiver, hospital administrator—can take a shot at writing a great poem. I love the possibility that reading a poem written by *someone else*'s patient can give a doctor an epiphany about one of her own. I love that we can give people who labor in the healthcare trenches, or who are the walking wounded, a forum in which to share their uniquely personal hopes and fears. Most of all, I love that *Pulse* creates an e-community committed to speaking the truth—about our deepest losses, our highest triumphs and everything in between—with grace and grit.

Johanna Shapiro PhD

At first, the words "excellent" and "poetry related to health care" might seem an unlikely juxtaposition—but that is exactly the right description for the poetry that appears in *Pulse* every three weeks. It can, in fact, be seen as a perfect realization of the magazine's mission. *Pulse* is a magazine that features healing, first-person narratives of giving or receiving care; and you could argue that, in some respects, poetry is the most personal narrative there is.

A *Pulse* poem may come from the pen of a health practitioner, a patient or a family member. Not surprisingly, these poems of illness and pain (or sometimes, thankfully, a full recovery or cure) often display widely divergent points of view. The professionals' poems tend to make some reference to the authors' hard-won expertise and training; the patients' poems of course reflect *their* authors' equally hard-won perspectives on pain and illness. But whatever the poems' origins, they always share, and give voice to, a deep inner core of humanity.

With my fellow poetry editor, Johanna Shapiro, I have the enjoyable task of selecting the poems that appear in *Pulse*. It is a happy task, but not an easy one. The standards are exacting, and over time the submissions have increased in both quantity and quality, making our decisions more difficult—even, at times, wrenching.

In selecting poems, we look for skillful wordcraft, sharply observed and evocative imagery and a transporting sonority. (Poetry is, after all, about image and metaphor, sound and song—and poems are sound, image and form all at once.) We also seek to detect, underlying all of these virtues, the throb of a warm and feeling human heart.

And so we sift through each submission for its substance. Needless to say, this requires numerous readings. With some poems, one or two suffice; but with really strong entries, we find ourselves returning again and again. Good poems not only survive rereadings; they thrive on them. With a good poem, repeated reading acts as a kind of hurricane, swirling through the fronds of words, shaking them free of their accustomed meanings, allowing them to offer up multiple other meanings and further surprises.

Consider, for instance, the poem "Morphine, Pearl Harbor" by Ann Neuser Lederer. She writes of the nurses that "they make their gentle mark" on the dead, the dying and those who have received the morphine. This lovely poem's meaning can be read in many ways. A mark can simply be a mark, a signature or sometimes a scar; in this poem, it is certainly also a method of creating recognition of triage and caregiving. One recalls how, in the *Odyssey*, it is Odysseus's old nurse who is the first to recognize him by his scar.

Only by this kind of scrutiny can we intuit or divine the kind of experience the poet aims to convey—and whether he or she has pulled it off. A single word set within an adequate space, and with just the right sound and depth of meaning, cuts immediately to the heart of the poet's message, and to the heart of the reader. With poetry, less is indeed more. And in the hands of a wordsmith, nuanced words, sounds and format can convey the author's experience subtly but exactly. The more indescribable and elusive the experience, the greater the challenge for the poet—but the greater the potential, too, for a truly compelling poem.

Stacy Nigliazzo's "Chirality" is an example of such rich, delicately layered allusions and associations, starting with the poem's title, a word signifying "the quality of some objects that cannot be superimposed upon their mirror images." The author goes on to use the image of the mirror to create reflection upon reflection: "I see myself, always/through a stark looking glass/the fun house view of my own face/reflected in the eyes of my patients...." Rereading this poem allows the reader to see the back of the mirror as well as its front, the patient's view as well as the nurse's, the micro as well as the macro.

This quicksilver flexibility of image and language makes poetry an exquisitely apt medium in which to communicate aspects of the world of health care; the field abounds in those urgently important yet undefined moments that poetry can capture so beautifully.

As a nurse, I can testify that we in the medical, nursing and allied professions live through countless such incidents. Many of our successes and near-successes are subtle and not easily described in the language given to us (forced onto us, dare I say?) by our medical and nursing education.

Meanwhile, on the other side of the stethoscope or the hospital bed, patients and their loved ones also experience such moments—moments that would remain inarticulate and indescribable unless expressed in poetry.

The poems that Johanna and I receive are a delight to read, and the process of savoring them and selecting some for publication has been the biggest joy of my experience with *Pulse*. And now the readers who have shared my pleasure in *Pulse*'s more recent poetry will have another medium in which to enjoy it—this second *Pulse* book, which (unlike the e-zine) can be touched and held, read and reread, put on the shelf and then taken down again for another reading.

Like the poetry and stories it contains, the book can be experienced on many levels. You can read it to enjoy the music of image, sound and form; you can read it to gain insight into another person's experience of illness or health. However you interpret it, you'll come away enlightened, touched and inspired; for *Pulse* is a textbook for the heart, mind and soul of anyone who has given or received care.

Judy Schaefer RNC MA

spring

Breaking Bad News

Paul Gross
4/24/2009

Bad news is like a lump of red-hot coal that lands in your palm—and that you can't let go of, no matter how badly you'd like to.

I was tossed the burning coal more than twenty years ago, when I was thirty years old and fit as a fiddle. Or so I thought. I also happened to be a first-year medical student, having my head filled with facts large and small about the human body.

Then something started to go wrong.

The first inkling came when I had to excuse myself from a two-hour seminar because of a sudden urge to pee. No big deal...and yet something about its urgency bothered me. The next time the seminar met, I took the precaution of urinating beforehand.

It didn't help. The same painless urgency interrupted the session once more. What was up?

Before long, I found myself using bathrooms a lot—in fact, more often than anyone I'd ever met. Within weeks, a one-hour class exceeded my endurance. So did the bus ride to school. And I certainly couldn't make it through the night.

Then the thirst began. A raging, playground-in-the-summer thirst that had me running back and forth from my desk to the kitchen, filling tumbler after tumbler with water or orange juice as I tried to study anatomy.

Clever fellow, I wondered whether it was the drinking that was causing the peeing. One night, to see what would happen, I went to bed thirsty. It didn't help.

Nowadays, as a doctor, I know that such symptoms mean only one thing. But back then, I couldn't assemble the disjointed facts I was learning into a clear picture. I assumed there could be a million causes for my symptoms, most of them treatable.

There was one piece of inside information that I chose to ignore as it flitted in and out of awareness: a cousin in his early twenties who'd developed an unquenchable thirst during a car trip—and landed in a doctor's office, where he was handed a diagnosis of diabetes, juvenile onset, and put on insulin right away.

When I thought about my unfortunate cousin, I wondered whether he had to inject the insulin directly into his veins, like a drug addict.

Luckily for me, I knew that I couldn't have diabetes.

How did I know? Because I was healthy. How could a person as healthy as me have diabetes? The logic seemed airtight.

The night that I had to use the bathroom five times, I finally decided to see a doctor. For some reason those five visits exceeded a critical threshold and convinced me that I needed help.

I had the good fortune to be covered under a student health plan whose office was in a red-brick building a few blocks from campus. An elevator took me up to a hallway, then I entered a waiting room.

Behind a sliding-glass window sat a graying secretary named Gladys, who greeted me and told me the doctor wasn't in. But after hearing my story, she made a call and described my symptoms over the phone. She listened, nodded and hung up.

"The doctor wants you to leave us a blood sample and come back tomorrow," she said.

The next day, I returned to the brick building filled with hopeful anticipation, like a pilgrim in search of salvation—or a patient fully expecting a cure.

I entered the small, empty waiting room. Gladys looked up from the open sliding window. And that's when it happened. Before I could sit down or even register the look of concern on her face.

"Oh, Paul," she said. "The doctor's not here again today; she wants you to see a physician downstairs. It looks like you have a problem with diabetes."

There it was. In my palm. The burning coal. Hot. Searing.

Ouch.

After leaving the building, I made a woeful, shell-shocked telephone call to my girlfriend. Together we tried to process this bombshell.

A few days later I was hospitalized, learning how to inject myself with insulin (I did not, thankfully, need to hit a vein, just pierce the skin) and how to test my own blood sugar. I began to contemplate my new life—totally dependent for survival upon insulin, syringes and blood-testing gadgetry.

All of that made me sad. But the thing that stung most was the way I'd been told the news. I felt angry at Gladys, though I later came to know her as a nice person who'd been thrust into a role she wasn't trained to play. I felt mad at the invisible Dr. X, who'd diagnosed and discharged me through an intermediary. Finally, I felt mad at myself because I might have complained, but never did.

Now, twenty-five years later, I'm a physician who on occasion delivers bad news to patients. Sometimes it's really bad, like cancer. Sometimes it's emotionally devastating, like a sexually transmitted infection in someone who believed that her partner was faithful.

Oddly, I like being the one to give the news. Not because I enjoy inflicting pain. Rather, it's a form of repair. It's a chance to rewind the clock and imagine someone taking care of me the way I wish a real doctor had.

Because of my experience, I know the impact of bad news badly delivered. And I know how long the memory lingers.

When I teach residents how to deliver bad news, I think of a cookbook recipe. Close the curtain or door. Make sure everyone is seated. Ask the patient what he or she thinks might be causing the symptoms in question. And then, making eye contact, say some version of, "I'm afraid I have some bad news to share with you..." If it feels right, touch the patient with a comforting hand.

Then comes the most difficult part: Say nothing. Wait for whatever comes. Silence. Tears. Or an impatient "So what do we do next?"

Teaching residents how to break bad news isn't much of a stretch for me. All I need to do is remember what it felt like—and what I myself wished for—when someone tossed me the burning coal.

_____

About the author: *Paul Gross is founding editor of* Pulse—voices from the heart of medicine.

Does the Buddha play pool?

Lenora Lapidus
5/1/2009

Come Medicine Buddha
Come shine your rays upon me
Penetrate deep within my body
To quell my queasy stomach
And soothe my aching bones.

Let those golden arrows
Shoot deep within my frame
Extinguishing the round tumors
That live inside of me.

Like a pool cue poised and ready
Aim straight for the triangle
Number 6 in right side pocket
Red 4 to far left corner.

Knocking away each colored ball
Dropping steadily into the pockets
Clearing away the hard assortment
Until only white and black remain.

The 8 ball holding fast
White blood cell gearing up.

And, then, a final shot—and POP!
No more colored balls
The table's cleared.

About the poet: Lenora Lapidus is an attorney and the director of the Women's Rights Project of the American Civil Liberties Union. She litigates in courts throughout the US and engages in public-policy advocacy before legislatures and executive-branch agencies as well as in international human-rights forums. Her work addresses employment discrimination, violence against women and educational equity for women and girls. In addition to her legal writing, Lenora has written and read poetry for many years. She lives in Brooklyn, NY, with her husband and daughter.

About the poem: *"This poem was written shortly after I was diagnosed with metastatic breast cancer that had spread to my bones. It was one of several poems that I wrote during this time. I found the process of writing poetry very therapeutic."*

Each Day, same story

Jennifer Reckrey
5/8/2009

Editor's Note: During her first year as a family-medicine resident in New York City, Jennifer Reckrey recorded some of her experiences as a brand-new doctor.

I have been his primary doctor for the entire three weeks he has been on the hospital floor. Sometimes he drives me crazy. Once or twice I've asked my senior resident to take over for a bit so I can hide out, catch my breath and try to get some of my other work done. Yet despite his daily demands and my hours of exasperation, I have never felt this connected to a patient before.

Over these weeks, I have watched his health slowly but steadily deteriorate. He first came to the hospital because his home oxygen wasn't helping as much as usual when he got short of breath while walking. A week later he needed his oxygen whenever he felt anxious. Now he's short of breath all the time. Without a face mask constantly pumping pure oxygen, his skin turns ashy purple and he slowly becomes agitated, then delirious.

When I got to work this Sunday morning, the night team told me that overnight he had refused to wear the oxygen mask for hours at a time. Now he was sleeping with the mask in place while an aide sat watch, but I knew it wouldn't last.

Then the call came. He was off oxygen and quickly slipping out of control: He had just thrown his breakfast tray at the aide.

Coming down the hallway, I could hear him screaming. From the door, I saw his arms flailing as he fought to pull himself out of bed. His eyes were wild, and though he looked right at me, there was no recognition. I inched closer, not sure what would happen if I got in his way, but afraid that he might throw himself onto the floor if I didn't stop him.

All at once he lunged towards me and grabbed my arms. He pulled me close, wrapped his arms around my waist, burrowed his head into my belly and began to sob. The embrace was hard and awkward: me standing, him teetering on the edge of the bed. I wanted to pull away, but his grip was too tight. Entwined with him like this, I suddenly felt overwhelmed. I wasn't a friend, but I didn't feel quite like a doctor either.

After a moment, I managed to grab his left hand and twist him away a bit. Though his right arm was still locked like a vise around my waist, his head now pressed against the bulge of papers in my lab-coat pocket. I fumbled for his oxygen mask and eased it slowly onto his face. His gasps turned to breaths, and through the tears he began to speak, first in jumbled words, then more clearly.

"I saw her dead. And I saw you dead. What is happening? What happened? You were all dead. And I was dead, too."

With time and oxygen and deep breaths, his color returned a little. His eyes began to focus again, and the crowd that had gathered to help drifted back out of the room. He slowly let go of me and crumpled, muscle by muscle, back into his bed. Still frightened, he begged me not to leave him alone.

I knew that there was no reasoning with him. I had already tried. If logical explanations had been enough, he would have agreed to take the right medications weeks ago. He would have followed up with the right doctors years ago. And he wouldn't have neglected his health in the first place. But things were what they were. All I could tell him was that, yes, I would stay for a while.

I pulled a chair next to his bed and sat silently, knowing that this gloomy calm was a temporary one.

Staying is the easy part.

At that moment, it feels okay to have nothing to show—no tangible improvement—for the time I've invested in this patient. At that moment, we're simply stuck with one another for a little while longer.

At that moment, I let go of my need to see things get better—and realize that, most of the time, things just get different.

About the author: *As a family-medicine intern in New York City, Jennifer Reckrey wrote weekly reflections about her experiences as a new doctor. "Even now I am haunted by my memories of this patient. He lived and then died (only a few weeks after I wrote this) by his own rules. His premature death was tragic, but the honesty with which he approached his life was admirable."*

counting cards

Alexandra Godfrey
5/15/2009

Once again, I see a still heart. As I stare at the fetal monitor, I search for signs of life. The screen flickers; my son's heart does not.

The last time I saw him, he looked happy—content in his life-bubble. As he turned somersaults, he waved at me. I had thought he was saying hello, but I realize now that he was waving goodbye.

Soon I must deliver his still form into the world. My labor will be difficult—his cries exchanged for my tears; his body, small and membranous, fitting into my one hand.

This is not what I had envisioned. I had dreamt of my son's vitality, not his mortality. I contemplate the suffering—is there no way to tally up the trauma?

For the third time, I am faced with the loss of a child, and experience is not making it any easier.

When my first child was born, he too had a still heart. As he was rushed away, I was asked to give him a name. I called him Ben.

Life almost evaded him. Ben was born with a complex congenital heart defect that affects one baby in ten thousand. Without emergency cardiac surgery, the defect is lethal. I did not expect my son's birth to herald his death. I could not make sense of it—beginning and endings existing together, creating dimensions beyond my scope.

I'd thought that I had laid the foundations of his future so well, but the path before us buckled under the weight of my son's oxygen-starved cells. My dreams of life had been reduced to a house of cards. As I watched the doctors perform CPR on my son, I felt bewildered—fifteen compressions asking why, followed by two breaths of silence.

Ben came back to life. He remained blue, but his heart had a rhythm, and the ventilator breathed for him. An expert in pediatric cardiology tore a hole in my son's heart—a procedure crucial to bypass the defects that were killing him.

Students, residents and fellows marveled at my son's aberrant anatomy. His great vessels were reversed, his valves thickened and narrow, and his only coronary artery abnormal.

For the scholars of medicine, he was a fascinating case. For me, he was a lesson in suffering. I saw a small body broken—veins punctured, dreams shattered, love insufficient to heal the hurts.

Ben's cardiac defects would demand the skill of a thousand surgeons blended together and developed through time: a series of incisions and sutures born of countless errors and successes and honed into a single perfect operation. The surgeon drew me pictures, the nurses gave me hope, and my friends sent beautiful cards without messages of congratulations.

On the twelfth day, the surgeon cracked my baby's chest open, stopped his heart mid-beat and then began to redirect the flow of his life's blood.

His surgery took hours. I ate tasteless muffins, drank insipid coffee and lit a candle in the chapel. I was instructed not to linger by the operating theater or ICU. Apparently, it makes it worse. So I resigned myself to the waiting-area fish tanks, paintings by Monet and rocking chairs placed by windows that framed the living. I watched a man pick up his child and a mother push a stroller along the pavement. I wondered if I would ever do the same.

Before my son left for surgery, I had tried to ask if he would die. I'd played with all the usual euphemisms, hoping the doctors would catch my question, but they never seemed to hear. I wondered if my words had gotten lost in the breeze of the ventilator, or maybe tangled up in the myriad lines that sustained my son's life. Sometimes now I wonder if they were buried under the piles of textbooks that speak only of curing

As it was, Ben survived the surgery. Against all the odds, my blue baby came home.

Years later, I lost a pregnancy at eight weeks. This time, I was not too surprised. Many pregnancies are lost in the first trimester, and I knew that I was not exempt from that rule. I grieved for my lost child, but I believed that my next pregnancy would be safe. I'd had my share of loss, I felt; life would not make me suffer any more.

Now, as I look at the ultrasound screen and see yet another still heart, I know that there are no safety nets; one disaster does not shield you from another. We can understand and play around with the variables, but we are never protected from that chance statistic…that one-in-ten-thousand anomaly.

The doctor offers me five days to keep my son with me. Then I must deliver him.

When I leave the hospital, I see people smiling at my rounded belly. One lady asks, 'When are you due?"

I say, "In five days."

My son and I go home together. I sit in the rocking chair in my bedroom, look at the Monet that is now on my bedroom wall, then in my heart and mind I paint for him a window adorned with angels.

There's a lot to be said to one's son who is already dead.

I suspect that over the next week the mailbox will again fill with beautiful cards without congratulations. Maybe, after all, these cards are the best measure of my suffering.

About the author: Alexandra Godfrey is a physician assistant in emergency medicine. "I have always had a deep love for language. I adore playing with the spaces between the words; there's so much room for creativity and expression. The death of my baby son moved me from reading the work of others to writing my own stories. My son Benjamin is doing well. Doctors, students and fellows still marvel at his cardiac abnormalities. Ben's future remains uncertain, but for now he enjoys a full and happy life. His brilliance is highlighted by his difficult beginnings. This is our privilege, and I am grateful."

failure to thrive

Daniel Becker
5/22/2009

My matched set of nonagenarians

is almost two hundred years old
and nearing escape velocity.
They are failing to thrive with a vengeance.

They have outlived everyone
except the powers of attorney
for whom they are a source of consternation.

Their constipation is prune-proof.
They scratch where it itches till it bleeds
and call on me to staunch the bleeding.

They can't recall our earnest conversations.
Adult Protective Services
elicits

their indignation reflex. They ready, aim
and fire
their walkers at the social worker.

Pride goes before their falls.
They hoard.
In their home every room is attic.

Neither odor nor order matters.
Thank goodness you're here they say
and then berate me.

It's true.
I don't know what to do.
I meet the lawyer at the bedside.

I meet the notary at the bedside.
We arrange for the funeral home
to call me at home.

By the end their ashes plus the urn
will weigh more than they did.
The wind always knows what to do.

About the poet: Daniel Becker practices and teaches general internal medicine and palliative care at the University of Virginia School of Medicine where he also edits the online journal Hospital Drive. In August he teaches at the Taos Writing Retreat for Health Professionals.

About the poem: "This poem includes bits and pieces of a few thousand years of nonagenarians who have stubbornly and gleefully taught me what is best for them. I'd like to dedicate it to them and to the future nonagenarians now gracing my waiting room."

piece of work

Jennifer Frank
5/29/2009

"You're a real piece of work!" he spat at me. He was a patient named Martin; I was the supervising physician, trying to role-model for a second-year resident how to conduct a difficult conversation with patients like this.

So far, not so good.

At first glance, Martin seemed an ordinary-looking older man, with close-cut gray hair and plain-framed eyeglasses. But I was struck by his scowl—he was expecting an argument, perhaps because during his interview with the resident he'd already encountered some pushback.

He'd brought a long list of laboratory tests that his biofeedback "doctor" had instructed him to get, saying that his fatigue and other symptoms were caused by "adrenal dysfunction."

I scanned the list—thyroid, blood count, chemistries, vitamins, adrenal function. *Testing for vitamins*, I thought. *Are they kidding?* Normally, we test for only a small handful of vitamins; would our lab even know how to test for the others?

Outwardly, I tried to look neutral. "If I order a lot of tests, it's statistically very likely that one will come back abnormal," I said. "That may not indicate a real problem; it could only mean that you'll end up having more tests."

"I want all of them. That's what my doctor said," Martin replied.

"Which vitamin was your practitioner concerned about?" I inquired.

"All of them, and minerals too," he said.

Taking a deep breath, I tried to explain the difficulty of testing for every single vitamin and mineral. Martin sat scowling, then erupted with his "piece of work" comment, following up by accusing me of being a "pill pusher" with links to the pharmaceutical industry.

I wasn't thrown by his verbal abuse, having seen my share of angry, slightly nutty patients. Mentally, I buttoned up my austere white coat, then responded that I wasn't pushing any medications, and that—unlike his bio-feedback practitioner—I had no financial interest in the treatments I pre-scribed. Furthermore, I added, no one had forced him to seek our help.

"You're the only one who can order the lab tests," he retorted. "That's why I'm here."

Finally I said, "I've explained which tests I feel comfortable with, but I won't order every single one." I couldn't help tossing in that there was a reason why his biofeedback practitioner wasn't allowed to order labs or write prescrip-tions. Then I left the room.

Later I commiserated with the resident: "I don't know why he bothered to come, if he thinks so little of us. Patients like that can be really frustrating." If Martin's complaints reflected anything, I thought, it was probably a mood disorder—not something organic.

I was surprised to learn, a few days later, that Martin's lab work had revealed chronic lymphocytic leukemia, a potentially deadly disorder.

My feelings ran the gamut, from dismay and guilt to near-indignation that Martin's fatigue was due to a real medical condition (one I would have tested for anyway if he'd come to us first). But I felt ashamed that I had belittled Martin for distrusting me, with my white coat and official title. Not only had my scorn damaged our relationship, past or future; it had diminished me in my resident's eyes, making me seem less professional and compassionate.

Now that the resident had to tell Martin his diagnosis and discuss possible treatments, I also realized that my exchange with Martin had compromised their relationship too. Maybe now Martin wouldn't listen to either of us.

In the days that followed, I kept turning the encounter over in my mind, like a loose tooth I couldn't leave alone.

Most of all, I had to admit, my professional pride had been stung. Martin's suspicion, his choice of an alternative practitioner and his overbearing attempts to exert control over our interaction had wounded me. But when I reflected on my own behavior, I ached even more: It was nothing to be proud of.

One of family medicine's challenges is the uncertainty that surrounds some physical complaints. Is someone's fatigue caused by cancer or by depression? How many tests do I order for a symptom that I'm pretty sure is related to emotional stress? When I forge a good relationship with a patient, we can then discuss the pros and cons of a potential intervention and reach decisions together—and it keeps each of us from feeling alone as we cope with the uncertainty.

My interaction with Martin had robbed us both of this relationship. Seeing no clear way to build rapport, I'd retreated to a comfort zone: being the medical expert. Then I was left trying to give a know-it-all explanation for a notoriously elusive symptom—fatigue. And when we did find a definite explanation for Martin's tiredness, my expertise wasn't backed up by a therapeutic relationship that could bring him into treatment. It made me realize that no number of "right answers" can substitute for forming a strong bond with another human being—a bond that enables you to provide care in every sense of the word.

Since that encounter, I've made a point of inviting patients to express their concerns and beliefs—and to question my recommendations. Some respond with the traditional "You're the doctor; you decide." Others take the opportunity to tell me what they really think about the practice of medicine.

I've become more open to my patients' beliefs, even those I consider off the wall or just plain wrong, and more willing to meet them halfway in negotiating what kind of care they'll receive. This approach helps them to feel better taken care of—and it allows me to mentally take off my white coat and feel like a true caregiver.

About the author: *Jennifer Frank is a family physician in private practice in the Fox Valley area of Wisconsin. "I've always enjoyed writing, but have turned more and more to the storytelling aspect of writing as a way to process difficult patient encounters and the feelings these evoke. I feel so fortunate to have the opportunity to learn from my residents and patients—they continue to challenge me to be a better person and doctor."*

TO MY LEFT

Anne Herbert
6/5/2009

I walk down the airplane aisle, scanning the rows. My eyes finally fall on 15F. My seat.

My nightmare.

This window seat means only one thing to me: someone to my left. A man, to be exact—middle-aged, reading the *New York Times* and snacking on a bag of peanuts. He doesn't notice as I shove my purse under the seat and sit down. My only thoughts are of blending in—with the other passengers, with the chair, with the plane itself. Anything.

My objective on this five-hour flight is simple and clear. It's the same one that I cling to almost every second of every day: to keep my left side hidden from the world.

Everyone has a good side—a more photogenic side, a certain way that they turn when taking pictures. I don't have a good side, but rather a "less bad" side—a side whose mere completeness is what appeals to me.

My left side charts the history of my birth defect. My severe underbite is an orthodontic byproduct of my cleft lip and palate. The scar under my nose records the surgery that closed my cleft lip. The scar on my hip commemorates a bone-marrow transfer from hip to mouth in second grade.

After a moment of going unnoticed, I feel the man staring. His stare digs into me, and I squirm.

In his eyes, my body has suddenly disappeared. All that's left is my profile, begging for scrutiny: nose, complete with scar; bottom lip jutting out farther than the top.

A damaged silhouette. Not like the beautiful black silhouettes you see framed in your grandmother's house. Not even like Alfred Hitchcock's portly outline—at least he is whole, unblemished.

The man to my left starts the airplane chat that everyone dreads. I don't want to answer, but I know that if I don't turn to him, he will end up staring directly at my left side.

If only I could show him a good side—present a better face to the world. But no matter which way I turn, someone is always to my left....

The paragraphs above capture a time in my life when my appearance dominated my thoughts.

I was born with a cleft lip. My very first operation, to close it, took place when I was three months old. I can't remember a time when I didn't have a scar under my left nostril.

The scar was never of much consequence to me when I was very young. Sure, I didn't like having countless appointments with my orthodontist and surgeon, but I honestly thought that all kids had to do this.

My parents never made it seem unusual. To this day, my mom says that she counts herself lucky: Although both of her children were born with minor birth defects, they didn't have any life-threatening complications or truly debilitating health issues. I constantly strive to embrace that outlook.

Inevitably, school was where I learned that my scars made me different. Don't get me wrong: Even there, I was lucky. I always had friends, and I was never picked last for kickball. But children are honest to a fault.

I became a master of evasion: I spent my youth skirting questions about my cleft lip—"What is that under your nose?"—that no adult would have the audacity to ask. In second grade, when I starting wearing a retainer, a classmate incessantly asked, "What is that? Why do you have it? Can you take it out? Can I see it?" She meant no harm, but it brought me attention that I in no way wanted. In fifth grade, a boy notorious for bullying asked me if a dog had bitten me in the face. Even though I knew he was a jerk, his words stung. In high school, when one or two friends asked about the bone-graft scar on my hip, I made up a ridiculous story about getting scraped on a fence when I was little.

It would seem that after two decades of acquaintance, my scars and I should have worked out our differences—perhaps even become chummy. You know, like when women who used to hate their curly hair embrace it and stop the daily blow-dry; or when the formerly embarrassing gap between someone's teeth becomes something "special" and "unique."

But this magical transformation hasn't been possible for me. My scars are a reminder of hard nights spent in the hospital. Of stitches being slowly, painstakingly pulled out by my surgeon. Of the six-week liquid diet I endured after my jaw surgery. So I still dislike my scars, and I certainly wish I didn't have them.

The most I've been able to do is to work out a truce. I realize that, like it or not, we're in a lifelong relationship, and after years of fighting, I want to make peace. So although I know that my scars will always be with me, I no longer let them monopolize my thoughts and actions.

Nowadays on my frequent trips from New York to California, I often sit in the window seat. I can go whole days without wondering, "Who's looking at my scar?" If a good friend asks me about it, I tell the truth. I even got up in front of sixty people during a public-health presentation and told them how I'd been born with a cleft lip and palate. We talked about organizations like The Smile Train, whose medical teams train surgeons in developing countries to perform cleft surgery.

No longer am I a master of evasion. Now I look straight at myself—and I let others look, too.

And *that* is liberating.

About the author: *Anne Herbert is a first-year medical student at Weill Cornell Medical College in New York City. A graduate of Stanford University, she first became interested in creative writing while taking Professor Lawrence Zaroff's class Medicine Through Literature.*

now a lightness

Fasih Hameed
6/12/2009

4:57 am, Sunday
This week went
from caring with hope
for a lucid patient to facing
reality in advocating sanity
to an insane extended
family to haggling with specialists
to giving up time
and again telling Mary
she was dying and then watching
her cling to her lost life like
everyone else to
finally withdrawing all care
except for comfort
and comforting the now lucid family
while the breaths became

                            distant

and the pauses

      prolonged
and everyone
cried, including myself,
when

      the last one

              left.

It was raining
when they called me. The family
said it just started, right before
the end. Like the sky had opened up

to let her in.

About the poet: *Fasih Hameed is a family physician practicing in Santa Rosa, California. When he wrote this story, he was completing a fellowship in integrative medicine for the underserved. He has dabbled in the creative arts all his life and is currently focusing on music (guitar/vocals/percussion/composition), poetry and building wooden surfboards. In medical school he worked with the art group Students Against Right Brain Atrophy, and he still organizes and attends peaceful anti-atrophy rallies whenever possible.*

About the poem: *"I wrote this poem as a resident, after guiding a patient and her family through a long and difficult journey towards a peaceful death."*

touched

Karen Myers
6/19/2009

"I can feel the life force leaving me," Mike says as he massages my legs with his rough, careful hands. He doesn't use oil or lotion like the other massage therapists. Just his sticky, Marlboro-scented fingers. I lie in my underwear beneath a green sheet. My bony shoulder blades and crooked spine press into the table, having long since lost their cushion of muscle.

"We're getting older," Mike says, even though we've barely reached forty. "Maybe that's why we're so afraid. We don't have the energy to fight like we used to."

Mike's eyes bulge like a bullfrog's. When I first knew him, I found them a bit frightening. His voice is raspy and deep. He has a fading tattoo on his left biceps and a ponytail that curls down his back. I met him at the massage school, where he was training to be a therapist and I was getting treatment for muscular dystrophy. I always thought he was quirky, and he talks too much, but his massages are cheap.

Since my diagnosis at age fourteen, when we first noticed a slight limp and a protruding shoulder blade, I'd spent most of my years ignoring my body. I pushed myself to work and play as hard as everyone else. I wanted to deny the disease that would cause a slow wasting away of the muscles throughout my body. By the time I hit thirty, my right arm was thin as a matchstick and could barely hold a dinner plate. A trip to the supermarket used up my stamina for the day. Stairs were harder to climb. My body was shrinking away. I moved to San Francisco, the mecca of alternative therapies, in the hopes that my dying muscles might come to life again. In the end, I found massage and bodywork the most beneficial.

"I can scare away animals with my eyes," Mike says as he moves my toes in circle formations. My ankles don't flex as easily as they used to. I swallow hard and try to relax. "There are these bees around my house, and if I take all my angry energy and focus it at them, they fly away. It works with people, too."

His anger, he tells me, is the only thing that keeps him going. He should be paralyzed by the disintegrating discs in his spine that cause him constant pain.

"I don't believe in God," Mike says as I turn onto my stomach. "There's no way there's a God. There's so much suffering by so many people." As I stretch out my legs, my fingertips brush against a hollow crevice formerly occupied by muscle in the backs of my thighs.

The night before, I'd been seriously praying. The kind of prayer where I actually speak out loud. The "Oh God, I can't handle this anymore, I don't know what to do, please help me!" kind of prayer. The muscles in my body were so sore, I thought my disease would finally knock me down. I'd been going to the pool and eating leafy green vegetables as my holistic doctor had recommended, but still fatigue enveloped me. Fear gripped me so tightly that I could barely breathe. Should I exercise more, exercise less, speed up, slow down, get more bodywork, get less bodywork, stop the vitamins or take more?

At 10:00 the next morning, Mike called me.

"Hey, Karen," he said. I hadn't spoken with him since our last massage, eight months earlier, but he didn't find it necessary to identify himself. "I'm in town doing massages, and somebody just canceled. I got a gut feeling I should call you. If you come over right now, I'll give you a session."

I know Mike is a little out there, but he's been a thread in my life—one of those people who emerges every once in a while, like a flare in a pitch-black night. He can meet me at my deepest points of despair and help me find the wisdom there.

"Feel that?" Mike says as he presses on the knot in the middle of my back. "That is the place that holds your breath. If you open that up, you'll release a lot of emotion."

Mike understands pieces of me in the same way that I understand pieces of him. His breath is caught in the same place of tightness; he talks about his own anxiety and depression as if it were mine.

"Take it easy on the exercise," he says. "Eat lots of ice cream, and have some fun. You're going to be fine." I laugh and feel a heaviness lift from my body.

I trust his words. Today, his wild eyes don't overwhelm me.

I get off the table, get dressed and meet Mike in the hallway. I open my wallet.

"No," Mike says, shaking his head. "Let's keep this clean."

I want to burst into tears. Mike is poorer than I am, and he won't take my money.

He reaches out and hugs me.

"It's really hard to be understood by 'normal' people," he whispers into my ear. "I know you understand me."

I wrap my arms around him and touch his broken spine.

About the author: Karen Myers is a freelance writer who has published many essays about her experiences living with facioscapulohumeral (FSH) muscular dystrophy. She is co-editor of the anthology My Body of Knowledge: Stories of Chronic Illness, Disability, Healing, and Life. *Visit her Web site at* www. CrackedBellPublishing.com.

summer

giving care

Ronna L. Edelstein
6/26/2009

When I was six, my family and I spent a week in Atlantic City. I loved the Boardwalk with its saltwater-taffy aroma and colorful sights, but I feared the pier that jutted far out into the Atlantic. One moonless night, my big brother bet me a bag of taffy that I couldn't walk to the pier's end by myself. Never one to back down, I accepted his bet. But the farther out I walked, the more frightened I got. It felt like one more step would send me off the pier's edge and into the bottomless black water. My parents rescued me by dashing to the end of the pier and carrying me back to safety.

I spent the next half-century living under two illusions: one, that nothing in my life would ever be as scary as that dark pier; and two, that my parents would always be there to save me. In school, when my Lilliputian classmates mocked my five-foot-eight-inch stature, Ma and Dad talked to me about inner beauty and strength. After the rice strewn along my wedding aisle disintegrated into sharp slivers of divorce, Ma and Dad gave me the financial and emotional support I needed to raise my son and daughter.

When after thirty-five years I returned to my hometown of Pittsburgh, I hosted Sunday-night dinners for my parents and ran errands for them. Yet they still saw me as their little girl; whether stocking my refrigerator or slipping mad money into my wallet, they made sure that I was okay. I found a balance between spending time with them and going out to dinners, movies and plays with my new circle of friends. Life was good.

Then, four years ago, like Alice, I tumbled into a topsy-turvy world. My eyes finally saw what my heart had refused to acknowledge: Ma was losing her mental edge. No longer was she the formidable woman who'd kept a spotless house and worked at a children's furniture store. And Dad, on our long walks, was leaning more and more on his cane and my arm for support.

My parents, once my constant caregivers, now needed me to be theirs.

As a result, I've spent the past four years feeling as if I'm once again tottering towards the pier's end—this time with no rescue in sight. To make room for Ma and her dementia and Dad and his aging, I willingly relinquished the starring role in my own life, feeling that as they had so willingly given to me, I should give to them.

Being an educator, I initially tried to embrace caregiving as a learning experience: Trying to feed Ma pieces of chocolate-chip cookies, I immediately halted when she whispered, "I can feed myself"—reminding me that, even with dementia, she was still my mother, not a child.

I quickly realized that caregiving can be a harsh teacher. I had to make difficult decisions: placing Ma in an assisted-living facility; giving up my apartment to move in with Dad.

And day-to-day caregiving, I discovered, is a powerful mix of deep satisfaction and profound irony. As Ma passively let me change her dirty diapers and urine-soaked bedsheets, I found myself resenting the distasteful tasks and mourning the feisty, capable woman I'd so admired. And when she mistook me for her sister, or a total stranger, I couldn't rationalize away my hurt. Other times, we would enjoy a moment of grace when she held my face in her hands and called me by name.

When Ma died in my arms in March 2007, a part of me rejoiced that she was finally at peace. Another part wondered if I myself could ever find peace, and whether I'd done my very best for her.

Life with Dad—physically weakened but mentally sound at ninety-three—offers its own highs and lows. Often my one and only wish is that our life together would never change. I love taking him to the mall for lunch or to the park for an afternoon of people-watching. Every night I massage his arthritic legs; every Saturday we travel back in time together, watching *The Lawrence Welk Show.*

Although Dad encourages me to spend time with friends, he gets despondent and frightened when I do make plans. So I've had to ask friends' understanding for my dwindling availability, and my once-full calendar is now rows of blank spaces.

I loathe my friends' emails describing "must-see" movies or plays that I probably won't. And I resent my brother when it feels like he's able to visit Paris and London but somehow can't manage the twenty-minute drive to see Dad.

At night I toss and turn, as if trying to claw my way out of this rabbit hole that has swallowed my life. I sometimes vent my pent-up feelings with a therapist-friend or use my iPod music or treadmill walks to calm down. But, like a child worried that stepping on a crack will break a parent's back, I try to avoid complaining, for fear that some avenging angel will take Dad from me.

And time, like Alice's White Rabbit, keeps racing ahead.

Sometimes I fantasize awakening one morning to discover, like Alice, that my experiences have been a dream, and that Ma and Dad are their old selves again. But deep down I know that, instead, someday I'll find myself truly alone at the end of the pier.

When that happens, I hope that the lessons I've worked hard on as a caregiver—patience and perseverance, acceptance of unplanned moments, tolerance of change, kindness towards myself and others—will stick with me and help to steady and support me as I step forward into my new life.

About the author: Ronna Edelstein is a teacher and a lifelong student, a daughter and a parent, a caregiver to her ninety-six-year-old father and a recipient of others' care. As a part-time faculty member at the University of Pittsburgh's English Department, Ronna works as a consultant in the Writing Center and also teaches Freshman Programs, which introduces students to the university and the city. Her fiction and nonfiction works have appeared in New Slang, a New Literary Voice by the Women and Girls of Pittsburgh; Quality Women's Fiction; SLAB—Sound and Literary Artbook; The First Line Anthology; The Road to Elsewhere, Visiting Elsewhere, *and* When We Are *(all three by Scribes Valley Publishing)*; AARP Bulletin; Healthy Roots *(Forbes Health Foundation and Hospice)*; The Jet Fuel Review; Writer's Relief; Ghoti Online Literary Magazine *and the* Pittsburgh Post-Gazette. *Ronna dedicates this story to Dad, Ilana, Jonathan and, in memory, Ma.*

The Limits of Medicine

Frances Wu
7/3/2009

I can not change the color of the sky.
The texture of the rain, the distance of a star
must needs be fixed by ancient ritual
unaccepted by our modernity.

I can not change the length of your night.
The number of hours, the days of your life
are set by stern fate, impassive to sighs,
unsympathetic, and cold to your plight.

I can not count the breaths that are left.
Day into day, year into frightened morn,
only you, in your heart can know
the obscurity of the sand that now sifts.

I can not make a single tear move;
Its salt will wend its way to the earth
that calls with an irresistible force,
one that will not soon leave off.

I have been roundly trounced
by movements and thunderings greater
by far than my hand's grasp;
and for their final victory, I apologize.

About the poet: *Frances Wu is assistant director of the Somerset Family Medicine Residency Program in Somerville, NJ, and teaches at New Jersey Medical School/ UMDNJ and Drexel University College of Medicine. "My passions include caring for my patients as if they were members of my family; teaching family medicine, bioethics and patient safety to medical students and residents; and compressing my work into a half-time schedule in order to fit in the other important things in my life: I take care of my two sons and husband, volunteer for the Human Rights Clinic of the nonprofit HealthRight International, lead a neighborhood poetry-reading club and sometimes participate in National Novel Writing Month, which* takes place every November. Poetry writing is my way of savoring the moments of life that shape the soul."

About the poem: "I wrote this poem when confronting my aged father-in-law's slowly declining health. I am a family doctor—not his—but I certainly felt helpless in the face of his inexorable illness."

The save

Dan J. Schmidt
7/10/2009

I started medical school thinking I wanted to be a family doctor—someone who could work in a small town and deal with whatever walked through the door. But in our third year, when we received our first taste of clinical medicine, I found my surgery and ER rotations exciting. I was at our state's major trauma center, and I loved it. Fixing things gives me a thrill—and the power to save a life is even more alluring.

Each "save" felt like a miraculous triumph. Take the nineteen-year-old visiting Australian, stabbed in a random street altercation, his blood pressure dropping as fluid accumulated around his heart. Right there in the ER, he had his chest split open and his right ventricle patched by the very cool chief surgery resident.

But after several weeks of 5 am surgery rounds and every-third-night call, I started to feel a nagging sense of unmet need, both my own and the patients'. To me, it seemed that the specialized care we were giving was excellent but fractured: No one was responsible for the whole person.

It was 8 am during my third week of the rotation. The third-year resident had led us medical students through our rounds, and there'd been time for some drug-rep doughnuts before we headed down to the ER. At the nursing station, we joined those who'd been on call the previous night and were sharing their war stories.

"You shoulda seen what we just got!" said one of the students.

A twenty-something guy had come in with a near-amputation. "He cut off his arm with a Skilsaw!" (the powerful circular saw used by professional carpenters and builders). "He's down in the OR now. Orthopedic surgery thinks they can reattach it."

After the descriptions of the bones, the x-rays, the blood loss, I asked one student, "Which arm?"

She frowned. She didn't know. I looked at the x-rays. It was the right.

I caught the gaze of a third-year surgery resident and asked, "Do you know how hard it is to run a Skilsaw left-handed?" (It's a lot harder than scissors. I knew: I'd spent a year building condos before I'd entered medical school.)

The resident nodded. This injury was no accident.

That evening I heard the orthopedic surgery team talking about how happy they were with their neurovascular and bone-plating work. It looked like the patient's hand would be saved. But they were aware of his psychiatric risks: He was being kept in restraints until they could get a "full psych eval."

The guy was in the post-operative ward; when I'd gone around to check on my patients, I'd seen him. Straight black hair. Intense gaze. Cold affect. Girlfriend sitting at the bedside, then leaving in tears.

The next morning, the psych team came by to evaluate him. They started him on an antidepressant, but thought that he was no risk to himself.

Coming back from lunch that afternoon, I heard stat pages overhead, calling the chief ortho resident to a "thrash" on the post-op ward. Hurrying down the hall, I saw a bed barreling towards me, pushed by three residents. A nurse knelt on top of the patient and his bloody sheets, pressing her hands hard against his arm as they steered the bed into the elevator.

"What happened?" I asked the senior resident.

"He pulled it off! All that work, and he just pulled it off!" he raged.

Before the elevator doors closed, I heard him say, "Damn if we're putting this back on again! He'll get what he wants!"

And off they went, back down to the OR.

I went to his room. There were fine blood spatters everywhere, and a big, dripping arc across the far wall. The Filipina housekeeper quietly mopped the burgundy-stained floor, shaking her head.

A technological success. A medical catastrophe.

We had treated this man's injury, reattached his limb, evaluated his psyche—but not one of us had tried to care for the whole human being. It seemed that our academic and specialized-care system had accomplished a wondrous feat of technological prowess, without creating a focus that could actually heal the patient.

Standing amid the gory mess left by a man I didn't know—a man who seemingly wanted *not* to be whole—I realized that I wanted to treat the whole person.

So I decided to stick with family medicine and left trauma and surgery behind.

A save still thrills me, although in family medicine they are thankfully rare. I get to keep my eye on the big picture. And I'm rewarded by a constant stream of quieter saves—the type 2 diabetic patient who loses fifty pounds, the alcoholic who's been dry for a couple of years now, the young single mother who's learning to raise her infant well.

These triumphs, bloodless but still lifesaving, keep me going.

About the author: After seventeen years of practicing full-spectrum family medicine, Dan Schmidt now covers small-town practices on the weekends. Married, and with four grown daughters, he also fixes old cars and remodels houses—yes, sometimes using a Skilsaw. "I find that writing eases my need for reflection."

Story editor: Beth Hadas

millie

Edgar Figueroa
7/17/2009

Looking at Millie in her living-room-turned-hospital-quarters I can't help reflecting on the four years we've shared as patient and doctor.

We've come a long way since our first visit. I was an inexperienced resident; she was a wiry woman who looked to be in her late sixties but was actually fifty-three.

She'd sat back and stared at me, sizing me up.

"You know I have kids that are older than you?" were her first words.

I wasn't sure if she was complimenting me on my youthful looks or expressing uneasiness at having me as her doctor. I smiled, blushed, quickly refilled her prescription and asked her to follow up.

Over time, I grew quite fond of Millie; seeing her name on the schedule always sparked feelings of pleasant anticipation. She, for her part, somehow grew to trust me, and the health-center staff learned not to argue when she insisted on seeing only "my doctor." At each visit she would share more of her story: how hard she'd struggled for much of her life, raising three children as a single mother with little support and less money; how much she liked her cigarettes and the occasional drink.

Now Millie is dying, and I am trying to act like a country-style family doctor in New York City.

She lies in bed, rubbing at a lottery ticket—hoping to win a big prize so she'll have something to leave her children besides a meager savings account, medical debts and anguish.

"Every day I scratch four or five," she tells me, her words barely intelligible.

Three months back, she had come to me because she was losing weight and things just didn't feel right in her neck. I'd sent her to an ear-nose-and-throat specialist.

Confirming my suspicions, he found a tumor in her tonsils; it extended into her neck and the base of her tongue. Those little rubbery masses I'd felt in her neck were cancer-riddled lymph nodes, gradually coalescing into a solid mass that would slowly starve and suffocate her.

The specialist had laid out the treatment options for Millie, but she refused to be rushed into anything. She wanted to discuss things with "my doctor"—and, in the process, to convey her opinion of the ear-nose-and-throat man.

"That doctor is an asshole," she politely informed me. Although she respected his medical opinion, she said, she wasn't wowed by his bedside manner.

He'd glibly told her she should have aggressive surgery and radiation. But Millie found it an unappealing prospect to have her tongue removed, a hole cut through her neck, a plastic tube inserted into her windpipe and a feeding tube put into her abdomen. She decided to forego all surgery, chemotherapy and radiation. She was smart enough to know that, for her, it was a case of the treatment's being worse than the disease.

The specialist begged me to get her to listen, but Millie's mind was made up and there was no changing it.

Over the three next months, her neck masses grew larger. Eating became nearly impossible. And then came the pain...

A few days ago, recognizing that Millie was dying, I had talked with her about making arrangements. We'd agreed that she didn't have to go see "that asshole"—or any other—ever again. I'd arranged for home hospice care, which would keep her comfortable enough to enjoy her remaining time with her family. The hospice agency had brought in a nurse, a caretaker, a pain-management physician and all of the necessary supplies.

Now, seeing Millie in her living-room bed, I reflect that this set-up seems to be working well.

"Oh," Millie says, beaming: "I'm going to Atlantic City!" Her sister is organizing a trip for herself and a few girlfriends.

"And my daughter is writing to that...what is it called...oh yeah, the Wish Foundation, to see if I can go to Vegas."

Struggling to make out her garbled speech, I nod as if I understand every word.

I glance at Millie's frame, so tiny that it makes the hospital bed look gigantic. She has lost almost all of her body fat. She has to sit up at an angle; otherwise, her swollen tongue will flop back and block her airway, or her pooling saliva will send her into a coughing fit. We stare at the sixty-inch-screen television, bizarrely large for the room; an old movie is playing. I can't help noticing that some of the characters on the screen look bigger than Millie.

Sunlight streams in through the windows as a cool breeze blows across the room. The rancid smell of sickness and death that I've grown so accustomed to in the hospital is replaced by the smell of cigarette smoke billowing from an ashtray, and of the most wonderful soup cooking in the kitchen.

The buzzer rings. It's her brother, dropping off a paper bag filled with a fifth of whiskey and more lottery tickets.

"That's my doctor," Millie says proudly, pointing to me. I still blush when she says that.

"A doctor who makes house calls? In New York?" says her brother incredulously.

His hands grip mine as if we're old friends. Our eyes meet, and we bare our teeth in an awkward "I'm smiling, but only because I don't want her to know how sad I am" smile, then quickly turn away from each other as we sit down.

We all stare at the images on the screen. Millie fills a glass with whiskey.

"Want some?"

I politely turn down the offer. She sets her glass down on the end table, next to her bottles of morphine, her other medications and her cigarettes. If I didn't know better, I'd caution her about mixing alcohol with narcotics...but Millie has always called her own shots. There's no way I could ever change that.

I sit a while longer, enjoying my time with her—the way I imagine a country-style family doctor would. And when the time grows late, I turn to Millie and thank her for allowing me to visit.

Then I hug her goodbye, knowing it's for the last time, and walk out the door.

————————————

About the author: *Edgar Figueroa is a family physician and director of student health at Weill Cornell Medical College in New York City. "I had the great fortune to attend a residency program that trained us in narrative medicine and taught me to reflect, read and write to enhance my care of patients. Back then, I had to be forced to write about a patient who moved me; now I can't wait for the next opportunity to meet with my friends and share a story."*

wanting to be lovely

Kenneth P. Gurney
7/24/2009

Breast budding, spring leaves,
twelve, too young for babies,
she grasps her pillow to her belly,
the smell of the first crocuses,
the last cardinal's song
echoes from the hawthorn.
The lemons whisper in her ear
before she squeezes, rubs
the rinds on her damp skin,
her hand touches nylon,
lace, a mirror image river,
a windowless desire:
the first stirring of her fingers
between her thighs, the robins'
annual return becomes monthly.

About the poet: Kenneth P. Gurney lives in Albuquerque, NM, with his beloved Dianne. He edits Adobe Walls, *an anthology of works by New Mexico poets. His latest book is* This is not Black & White. *To learn more, visit* www.kpgurney. me/poet/Welcome.html.

About the poem: "The image of a girl wanting to be adult came to me nearly fully formed out of the artistic ether, and I painted what I saw with words."

invisible Thread

Donald O. Kollisch
7/31/2009

From: *Michael*
To: *Donald O. Kollisch*
Subject: *Serious medical update*

Don,

I can't say for sure why I'm writing to you, but you were such an important part of my life during the onset of my illness that I feel a strong desire to communicate with you.

The mysterious autoimmune disorder that was lurking in my body has finally had the decency to declare itself. Unfortunately, it is systemic sclerosis, also called systemic scleroderma, which means I'm facing a gradual but ultimately fatal process of skin, joint and organ degeneration.

It has hit my lungs, seriously affecting my breathing capacity, and has hit my digestive system also. Recently I was in the hospital for ten days because of serious digestive problems and an inability to eat. I'm now on intravenous nutrition, with a line in my arm. I can eat a small amount of food for pleasure, but there's a real question as to whether I can ever take in enough nutrition by mouth to get off the intravenous line.

My rheumatologist at DHMC is wonderful—a good, honest and very compassionate young doctor. She has been completely candid about what we do and do not know about the outcome of my illness. Actually, we know the outcome; it's the timetable that's in question. Next week I start a chemotherapy regimen: cyclophosphamide. There isn't a lot of evidence for its value in treating my condition overall, but it could slow lung deterioration enough to make a clinically significant difference.

So that's the bad news.

Here's the "better" news: I am not afraid of this. I don't love it, but I've always understood the concept of mortality. I think that the length of this illness, and its yo-yoing nature, have brought about great changes in me, for the better.

I know that the course of this disease is not pleasant, and I don't look forward to it. But my single strongest belief, taken from Buddhism, is that we can find meaning, purpose and value in life even in the midst of suffering. I truly believe this.

I am also very aware that I'm lucky to have a family around me as I go through this—a family whose members support one another. Not everyone has that. Over the past weeks, we've had many honest discussions about the situation. No one is in denial, but no one—myself included—is ready to hang up the black crepe paper.

I've been doing a lot of reading, thinking and journal-writing these past weeks, and it dawned on me that I was doing the work necessary to help me prepare to die—but also, far more importantly, I was doing the work to prepare to live with this. You prioritize; you ask what's important, what you still want to do. Now that teaching writing to my college students is no longer an option, I'm making writing a full-time activity, along with exercise (walking, tai chi, light hand weights).

As I said, I approach this without fear, but with a sense of purpose. I will let the doctors do what they can, and I will do what I can to make myself stronger. I have a very vital life force in me. It will run out, as it does for everyone, but meanwhile I get on with life.

I hope you don't mind, but I felt the need to share this with you.

Regards,
Michael

From: *Donald O. Kollisch*
To: *Michael*

Michael,

Thank you for writing. For reasons that I hope to articulate, it feels important to stay connected with you and to know what is happening.

When I go through an intense illness with someone, and hopefully provide some variety of help, whether it's diagnosis or therapy or guidance or simply being there, a bond forms between us. It can be a bond of shared gratitude—the patient grateful to me for whatever aid I provided, and I to the patient for opening up to me and sharing an intense human experience that even metaphor cannot convey. Sometimes the bond is a shared secret, dark or light—something very few are privileged to know. On rare occasions, a patient and I share the experience of a miracle.

This connection is what keeps me in medicine, because it is—for me— a unique and intense link that may fade with time but never extinguishes. As you and I traveled the path of your illness, this invisible thread connected us. I remember our talks about your strange symptoms, which came out of nowhere and retreated only reluctantly when treated with steroids. We agreed that your symptoms made no clear sense—and, grateful though we were that they'd receded, we also wondered about their underlying cause. I've carried your mystery within me since then, and it makes sense to me that you'd know this and reach out to complete the connection once more.

I apologize if this sounds mystical. I am not a mystic, but I am a doctor, and I believe that doctoring isn't just an intellectual exercise. Although I'm no longer formally responsible for your care—and I'm grateful to the rheumatologist for caring for you so well—I still care for and about you.

Thank you for so generously sharing your news and reflections with me. I hope that Judi and the kids are faring well—I've no doubt that they're wonderful in their support for you and for each other. And please let me know if there is ever anything I can do.

Regards,
Don

From: *Michael*
To: *Donald O. Kollisch*

Don,

Thank you for the meaningful and beautifully articulate response. I don't think you're being mystical, just human. (Although I believe there's more than a touch of the mystical in that.)

Throughout the different stages of my illness, when you were my doctor, I felt cared for both as patient and as a human being. We will keep in touch as things develop—and maybe even share the rare occasion you mentioned and experience a miracle together.

In the meantime, I continue to value the things in my life on a daily basis, and I'm doing a good job of living in the present.

Be well, and we'll be in touch,
Michael

About the author: Don Kollisch is a family physician whose first—and most influential—practice was in rural northern New England. The academic-medicine path then brought him to North Carolina, back to New Hampshire and to urban New York City. For fifteen years he's written short fiction based on the lives of his patients—farmers, loggers and the like. He has had stories published in regional magazines, online and in a print anthology. This piece is an edited exchange of e-mails with a former patient, Michael, who was pleased to see it published before he died.

Tug-of-war

Jo Marie Reilly
8/7/2009

As I teach first- and second-year medical students to take patient histories and to perform physical examinations, I always feel humbled and privileged—energized by their compassion, enthusiasm and facile, curious minds.

Occasionally, I feel particularly challenged—especially when I'm teaching a student who, though bright, is struggling to acquire some of medicine's basic skills. As we journey up the learning curve together, my responsibilities can conflict: As a teacher, I want to nurture an aspiring student physician; yet as a physician, I must ensure that patients receive appropriate care.

Now, sitting quietly in the corner of the room and watching a young medical student interview a county-hospital psychiatric patient, I begin to feel this tension.

"What brought you into the hospital?" the student queries nervously.

Small and reserved, she's quite a contrast to her patient—a burly, imposing middle-aged man, his body splattered with tattoos of birds of prey and firearms. He folds his arms tightly across his chest, and a large cross sparkles on his neck chain.

"It's when I tried to commit suicide on the bridge," he responds agitatedly.

There is a long, awkward pause. "So...what medication did you say you take?" she asks.

"I take respiridol. It's for my voices," he replies flatly.

The student clenches and unclenches her hands.

"What about drug allergies?" she asks. "Do you have any drug allergies?"

"No." He stares at her blankly.

"Alternative medical therapies?"

"No!"

She fidgets with her papers, looking through her history-and-physical book for the next question to ask this obviously disturbed man. Her eyes dart around the room's harsh, white walls, which are devoid of any mirrors and pictures. The stark surroundings make the interview even more intimidating.

As a seasoned clinician, I feel frustrated by the fumbling interaction unfolding before me. But as a teacher, I feel compassion for the student's discomfort with this emotionally fragile man and hope that she can find a way to connect with him. I continue observing silently.

The student locates a phrase on her mental-status sheet that seems to give her comfort.

"Your mood," she blurts. "How would you describe your mood?"

"Angry!" he shouts, picking furiously at some invisible specks of dust on his hospital gown and flicking them off with his fingers.

"Oh." She glances nervously past the bed-curtain to the guard watching curiously from his doorway post.

Okay, I think. It's time for an attending-physician rescue. I stand up and walk to the bedside.

"Mr. Adams, " I say, "tell me about the bridge. You must have felt pretty desperate to want to end your life."

He looks at me, relaxing a bit. "Yeah, I jumped from that bridge, but that fisherman pulled me out. Damn well near froze in that water."

Thinking that I've jump-started the interview, I nod to the student, who's been frantically scribbling down our conversation.

"I haven't asked you yet about your past surgical history," she stammers.

He simply looks at her.

"That's quite a story," I interject. "What made you so anxious that you wanted to jump from the bridge?"

"It was those voices again. When those voices come, it's all over."

The student looks at me; I raise my eyebrows encouragingly.

"How about immunizations? Did you receive your childhood immunizations?" she asks.

"Immunizations?" He looks at her strangely and begins to tap his foot against the bed. "What are immunizations?"

"Well, Mr. Adams," I say, "I actually think it'd be important to know more about those voices. Tell us about them. What do they tell you to do?"

"They tell me I'm worthless. They tell me to hurt myself." Looking distressed and ashamed, he gazes at the wall.

I pause, giving the student another opening.

"Let's see," she says, looking at her notes. "Did you ever do any military service?"

I look over at her again, trying to conceal my exasperation. Does she just not get it or what? Time to bring this painful interview to a close.

"Mr. Adams, you've been so kind to talk with us this morning. Your voices sound like they are very scary, and they cause you to do some unsafe things. How are your voices now?"

"They've quieted down since I got back on my medications," he says. "They're not telling me to kill myself anymore."

I nod. "I'm so glad that you're feeling safer now. We'll make sure the social worker gives you enough medicine so that when you leave the hospital you can keep your voices down. Can we do anything else for you today?"

"I just want to rest now. I'm pretty tired from all this talking," he answers, closing his eyes.

Out in the hallway, I turn to the medical student.

"How do you think it went?" I ask.

She glances at her notes, looking distracted. "I think it went pretty well," she says. "I got almost everything—but I did forget to ask him if he had a family history of diabetes."

I sigh inwardly. How can I give her feedback that is constructive and tactful? How much of her stumbling is due to her youthful inexperience and to the intimidating environment? With more maturity and less nervousness on her part, will her communication skills blossom?

The inevitable doubts set in. What is my role and responsibility as her teacher? How can I help her "get it"? What if, despite my best efforts, and those of my colleagues, she still cannot adequately listen and respond to patients? I dread the thought.

At such challenging moments, I think of my professional vows—the Hippocratic Oath's admonition, "Do no harm." As a teacher, I am called upon to do no harm to this hopeful, aspiring student physician. As a clinician, I must ensure that no harm be done to the patients she serves.

I must dig deeply for courage, patience and wisdom.

And so continues this tug-of-war.

_____

About the author: *Jo Marie Reilly is associate professor of family medicine at the Keck School of Medicine of the University of Southern California (USC), where she is co-director of the Primary Care and Community Medicine Program and assistant director of the Introduction to Clinical Medicine course. She is also a member of* Pulse's *Advisory Group. "Writing helps me connect with the power of humor, joy and compassion in the work that I do, and in doing so helps me balance my professional life and patient care with my personal life, which includes spending time with my family."*

johnny Doe

Yvonne M. Estrada
8/14/12

Policemen pose like plastic toy soldiers,
point rifle barrels in every direction,
ghetto bird's spotlight glints off helmets.
Ambulance allowed across yellow tape,
diesel engine grinds up the sharp grade.
In no moon you glow fish white belly up,
streetlamp casts mottled shadows,
your blood a preschool finger painting
smeared on sidewalk.
I am ordered to shear off your slick, soaked
jeans, to smash your chest, beat your heart
for you. Your arms extend savior-like,
needles are pounded into veins,
translucent bags held skyward
like offerings to a life-giving deity,
clear liquid bleeds in, your blood pours out,
three bullet holes versus six-minute
trip to emergency room. How old are you?
I think about my son asleep at home.
I wonder if *your* mother's at work.
I breathe deep, drive fast,
make the siren a prayer
too loud for your God to ignore.

About the poet: *An emergency medical technician for fifteen years, Yvonne Estrada currently works as an ambulance driver for the Los Angeles County Emergency Medical Services Authority. "I have always written poems, and my job naturally presents adventures and situations that need to be written about, stories that need to be told. My family and friends enjoy these stories, but it's also nice to have them read by people 'in the industry'." Estrada reads this poem and others at* www.guerrillareads.com *(she's No. 8).*

About the poem: *"Johnny Doe was inspired by the patient's being so young— only eighteen. At the time, my son was fourteen, and he was at home while I was at work."*

Looking for Respect

Ashrei Bayewitz
8/21/2009

This may sound strange, but I secretly looked forward to my colonoscopy.

I was excited to see the people in the colonoscopy suite—the receptionists, the nurses and my doctor. I knew that they would like me, because I would be brave and respectful. That's what's always happened since I was diagnosed with Crohn's disease ten years ago. During my multiple colonoscopies and countless doctor visits and other outpatient procedures, I invariably build up a rapport with someone, be it a doctor, nurse or staff member. I've always been a good patient, and now that I'm a second-year medical student as well, I can understand their work a little better. I expect them to sense my goodwill and to treat me in turn with respect and caring.

This appointment got off to a good start: The woman who registered me seemed nice and appreciated my interest in the pictures decorating her cubicle wall. And I wasn't just being polite—I really did like those black-and-white photos of old TV and film stars. She even had *The Honeymooners* up there! I also got along well with the first nurse—we shared a laugh about the trouble I'd had finding a quarter to pay for my locker.

But a few minutes later, my interview with the intake nurse took me aback. Staring at her computer screen, she recited a series of questions. Seated facing away from her in a gigantic reclining chair that seemed cemented in place, I couldn't turn around far enough to catch her eye. The nurse's lifeless, monotonous tones conveyed zero interest in who I was or what I had to say. I'd never felt so unimportant.

To make matters worse, people kept interrupting us. The first time it happened, I thought that something serious must be happening—maybe a patient was having difficulties, or the computer system had crashed.

No. It was lunch time. They needed to coordinate their takeout orders, and my nurse, it became clear, was the lunch organizer.

Sometimes coworkers called her out of the room (but not out of earshot); other times they conversed right in front of me. Eventually I got so used to it that I began letting her know when someone was waiting for her.

Still, I felt stung at receiving so little respect. Was I invisible? Couldn't their lunch plans wait a few minutes? Nevertheless, I swallowed my pride, reminding myself that healthcare professionals are people too, with needs of their own. Maybe my nurse had found that distancing herself from patients helped her to do a better job. When she expertly inserted my IV line, I felt I'd taken the right attitude. Our relationship wasn't very satisfying, but at least she had technical skills.

Soon I was called to the procedure room and introduced to my next nurse, who would actually assist with the colonoscopy. She seemed down-to-earth and likable, but that's when things really started to go wrong.

For one thing, she'd forgotten to put a bed in the procedure room. Then, when she did bring it in, she had me lie on it facing the wrong way. After we'd fixed these details, I heard someone down the hall talking excitedly about a "scholar." There must be some talented pre-med students shadowing the doctors that day, I surmised. Feeling a sense of kinship with them, and renewed self-confidence, I hoped that they would stop by my room.

When my nurse brought in the student, I waited eagerly for her to introduce us. Instead, she started helping the young woman to put on scrubs. And while that was happening, I learned that this "pre-med" student was actually a ninth-grader.

My pulse quickened, and my mind raced. Was I some animal in a zoo for children to gawk at? I was having a colonoscopy—the procedure where they stick a tube up your rear end. Couldn't they ask my permission before inviting a spectator?

Struggling to sound calm, I asked, "Does my doctor know that a student will be watching my procedure?"

My nurse didn't seem too pleased: I'd breached the unofficial patient's code of conduct. She blinked and said, "This is a teaching hospital," adding that patients should expect to be observed.

I knew that this was utter nonsense. As a patient and a medical student, I care deeply about the principle that a patient's dignity should be respected at all times. I felt ready to fight for this.

"It's probably okay," I said, "but it would have been nice if you'd asked me first."

"Patients can always refuse being observed if they wish," she retorted, contradicting her earlier statement.

All I wanted was an apology and an acknowledgment that they weren't allowed to coerce or take advantage of me. After some more back-and-forth, my nurse conceded her mistake. But the whole exchange left a bad taste in my mouth.

When my doctor came in and learned what had happened, he told me that I was under no obligation to be observed. Before I'd even finished nodding, the student was taking off her scrubs; a few moments later, she was gone.

Ironically, I still liked the nurse. I felt sorry for her that she'd been making mistakes, and I appreciated that she'd apologized for them. And when she started telling me about herself, I liked her even more.

She'd had a lot of experience in surgery, she confided, but was still fairly new to the colonoscopy suite. She'd felt that she had to let the student observe because her boss had requested it. Although it didn't excuse what she'd done, I appreciated her candor. It was as if we were meeting for the first time.

An hour or two later, I was waking up in the recovery area. Looking across the hallway, which looked blurry to me without my glasses, I saw someone walk by with a friendly wave and a smile. I can't say for sure, but I think I know who it was.

About the author: *Ashrei Bayewitz is a first-year resident in internal medicine at Winthrop University Hospital. He wrote this story as a summer intern at* Pulse, *when he was a second-year medical student at Albert Einstein College of Medicine. "I've been interested in writing since middle school, when I composed mock newsletters to celebrate the birthdays of friends and family. I am continually surprised by the interesting and sometimes humorous connections that I make while writing. Around the time that I chose to go into medicine, my love of stories evolved into a special interest in illness narratives. My honors thesis at Yeshiva University showed how these works can help doctors better relate to their patients."*

chris

Lisa deMauro
8/28/2009

My big sister Chris, fifty-five, had recently returned to her first career, nursing, when she wrenched her back one day while helping to lift a patient. After weeks of physical therapy proved unhelpful, her internist ordered some tests, which indicated that her back injury might signal something more sinister. She'd had a lumpectomy for a "stage 0" breast cancer five years earlier, and her doctor advised her to make an appointment with the newly appointed head of a brand-new cancer center nearby.

Chris and I were nine years apart—a difference that precluded any sisterly rivalry—and we'd always been very close. She'd occupied a central role in my life: first, as a playful second mother to me, then as my ideal of teenage glamour, and finally as a friend with whom I shared confidences about the joys and sorrows of grown-up life. When it became clear that she might be getting bad news, I needed to be with her, just as my parents did.

The three of us converged on the Pennsylvania town where Chris was living. We met her in the hospital lobby, hugged each other for long moments, then headed off together to meet with the oncologist.

Our collective mood was one of defiance born of family history: My mother had had a mastectomy in the distant 1950s, and my father had had surgery for thyroid cancer and was currently being treated for prostate and colon cancer. We were determined to be positive: Here we are! A family that faces down cancer! Survivors!

Of course, we were also terrified.

What we needed in that moment was a superhero—a confident, compassionate medical warrior who would stand between our family and the unthinkable possibilities, armed with brilliance, sensitivity and a detailed checklist of treatment options. What we got, inevitably, was a human being—one spectacularly ill-suited to our needs.

In a private sitting area we sat, huddled close for safety, and watched the white-coated oncologist approach. He greeted us with a smile that held no warmth, sat in a chair facing us and served up his news. In brief, factual sentences, as if summing up a case history in a textbook, he explained that Chris's back pain was almost certainly a symptom of breast cancer that had spread to her bones. There would be more tests, but he felt little doubt of their results.

It's a cliché to hate the person who delivers bad news, but this man left us no choice. Chris, divorced and with only her own income to rely on, asked just one question: "Will I be able to go back to work?"

The doctor smiled apologetically. "Did you want to go back to work?"

That's how we learned that she wasn't expected to recover.

A few days later, we met Chris's radiation oncologist. He was a gentle-seeming soul, perhaps even compassionate, but with no apparent concept of tact. He asked us to wait in a spare, corporate-looking conference room, and my parents and I exchanged numb looks as we hovered protectively around Chris.

The doctor came back in, placed a film on the lightbox, then beckoned us over. "Take a look," he said, pointing. "Here's your bone scan."

He might as well have said, "Here's your death sentence."

It's impossible to describe the hollowed-out, otherworldly feeling of that moment: We stared at images of a brightly lit miniature skeleton shot through with black dots. Tumors everywhere, too many to count—in the ribs, the thighs, the pelvis, the skull.

What did we say to each other then? Or in the car later on? I don't remember.

Chris was prescribed painkillers and scheduled for rounds of radiation. In the weeks that followed, she suffered terrible pain in her back and legs, along with violent nausea; she never went more than an hour without vomiting. My parents moved in with Chris to shop and cook, drive her to treatment and offer support. I obsessively searched the Internet trying to figure out *what to do.* I made weekly trips with offerings that I hoped would bring relief: ginger snaps, aloe juice, licorice, a microwavable pillow for the pain.

Weeks turned to months and Chris failed to improve—yet through all of this, the oncologist seemed weirdly disengaged. It was hard to get his attention; he seldom returned phone calls. It felt, in fact, as if he'd lost interest in her case. Clearly this wasn't going to be a success story. Perhaps, in his mind, he'd already moved on.

I feel deeply ashamed that through all those months we couldn't pull ourselves together and say, "Enough is enough." Finally, though, the oncologist pushed us over the edge. During a rare visit to his office, Chris began to vomit. For a second, he looked horrified. Then he laughed, patted her back and said, "She'll be all right."

That pat on the back did it.

We harnessed our outrage and started over: sifting through names, making calls, searching for someone who would accept Chris's insurance. When we did find a candidate, we had to gather Chris's massive medical dossier and lab reports and struggle to get her focused—most of the time, she felt too ill to leave the house—hoping all the while that the next doctor would actually know how to help.

Finally, we found one who did. My sister's "good" oncologist was a gentle, genuine, white-haired man who seemed able to read the situation and offer exactly what was needed. Before he did anything else, he listened: to Chris, to learn what her daily experience was like; to my parents and me, to learn what our concerns were and what we needed in order to offer Chris support. His first priority was determining why she'd been so nauseous. When he changed her pain medication, eight months of vomiting came to an end in one afternoon.

In choosing a course of treatment, he took his lead from Chris. He never required her to look farther than the next appointment, nor did he go out of his way to remind her that her time was limited. He seemed to feel that the quality of her life, rather than his expertise, was the most important factor in her care. He brought peace and calm to our family and helped relieve the shame and hopelessness that my parents and I had felt.

Almost four years after meeting her first oncologist, Chris died. I believe that the outcome would have been the same no matter who treated her. But I know that fleeing her first, inadvertently cruel, care providers to seek the care of compassionate people made all the difference in her day-to-day experience.

I have infinite respect for the intelligent, courageous people who make oncology their life's work. But I've seen that it isn't enough to be knowledgeable or technically proficient. My sister's experiences convinced me of the vital importance of finding a caregiver who understands how to give care in every sense.

Chris's first physicians were doctors but not healers. Her last physician showed us that, although Chris's illness couldn't be cured, she could still experience healing. And, in fact, this healing offered the deepest comfort to my sister and to all of us who loved her.

About the author: Lisa deMauro is a long-time freelance writer and editor and a recently minted school counselor. She has gotten to know something about death and dying through the long final illnesses of two close family members and a beloved friend. She believes there is something liberating—and loving—about making the effort not to push mortality off to the side, but to allow it to come into the room and be contemplated and discussed.

chemo patient

Geoffrey Bowe
9/4/2009

She tried
To imagine herself dead
As she lay on her bed
Staring at the ceiling
With chemotherapy
Seeping into her veins
But she couldn't
She could only think
Of her husband
And her children
And how they had laughed
When her hair had fallen out.

In order to die
Everything had to stop
Her heart
Her brain
The blood surging
Through her arteries
But she could not imagine it.
Everything
Seemed to be running so well.

She was not frightened of dying
But she had always
Looked forward to the future
And now it seemed
There may not be one.
It was not like her
To look backwards
So she carried on
Staring at the ceiling
And tried holding her breath.

About the poet: *Geoffrey Bowe has been writing poetry since he was sixteen and has written nursing poetry since he trained as a nurse, several decades ago. His work has appeared in two anthologies of writing by nurses (*Between the Heartbeats *and* Intensive Care, *both U of Iowa Press) and in* Nursing Standard *and* The International Journal of Healthcare & Humanities.

About the poem: *"While nursing a young woman on chemotherapy, I observed her deep in thought—but rather than ask her, I tried to imagine what she might be thinking. Suddenly on the cusp between life and death, but still very much alive, could she possibly be imagining death itself and thinking how much has really got to happen before anyone dies? Her heartbeat, so strong—as it should be in a young woman—would have to stop, as well as all that goes on in her brain. Surely this, I thought, would seem unlikely and distant to her, even in this situation."*

The Emaciated Infant

Paula Lyons
9/11/2009

The police had been called to the house by a neighbor who said she heard children crying and hadn't seen the mother in two days. It was the middle of a night in July, and the children's wails would have traveled through the project windows left open to catch cooling breezes.

Paramedics provided transport to the hospital, but the normally cynical and well-defended police were so outraged that they also came to the ER, where I was the resident on call.

The police came to find and punish those who had neglected this waif, but I also sensed that, despite their tough exteriors, they came also to vent their impotent rage and to seek reassurance that this tiny, dirty, appealing thing would live. Our hospital had no pediatric ER staff, and although I was only a second-year family-medicine resident, I was the senior "pediatrician" in-house. And so I needed information. How was the baby found? What diseases had she been exposed to? Why was she so starved? I chose the greenest member of the team, knowing that he would be the most talkative. And, as a rookie myself, I sensed a kindred spirit.

The young cop was trembling as he described the conditions in the apartment. "Three kids in the kitchen, all under eight years. The place was a wreck. There was moldy mac and cheese in a pot on the stove, and the oldest said that's what they'd been eating. We saw all these bottles with crusty milk lying around, but, like, no baby, you know? There was formula in open cans in the fridge, looked like a million years old. Roaches. I was in the bedroom, clothes everywhere, place stank, and I saw something moving under a pile of rags. Christ! I thought it was a rat."

He expelled a breath loudly, shaking his head, and turned to look yet again at the Emaciated Infant under the warmer, exposed in the revealing glare of the fluorescent ER lights.

Somalia comes to Baltimore. Huge pink belly and wispy thin hair. Inflamed, itchy-looking diaper rash all the way up to her nipples. Wizened. She mewled faintly. I'd never before seen a child this starved. I called the head of pediatrics at home and, bless him, he gave me good advice. I was afraid to feed her by mouth, but he said that in addition to IV fluids, antibiotics and warmth, a tiny bit of Pedialyte was allowable. The older children, less obviously damaged, had already been taken by Social Services and assigned to separate foster homes. I wondered if they'd ever see their sibs again.

Among the staff, there was an atmosphere of palpable rage, slightly softened by coos and aahs when the Emaciated Infant actually showed the will to suck.

What erases mother love? Cocaine. The cops had found razors on fragments of glass, and traces of white powder. They didn't wait for the forensics report before making their own judgment; they'd seen these telltale signs many times before.

Mother couldn't be located that night, and as for the father…who knew? The return address on an unopened Christmas card, discovered in the apartment by the rookie cop, led us to some relatives.

When the mother's parents arrived at the ER, the nurses punished them with the hard, bright, professional treatment, and with looks that chastised more harshly than words. They were prepared to hate any adult who they thought had known, or should have known, of the infant's plight yet had done nothing to save her.

The baby was named Victoria, her grandparents said. She was only four months old. Then, as these portly people in their sixties held each other and wept loudly by the warmer, oblivious to everyone but Victoria and each other, the staff visibly relented. The charge nurse brought them tissues and, with a snap of her wrist, drew the bed-curtain around us. I encouraged Grandmom to touch Victoria's matchstick arm, having noted with hope that the baby smiled and curled closer in response to touch.

Though the cops wanted justice (and vengeance), there was no one present to blame. Grandpop, limping with arthritis, blew his nose wetly and went outside to sit on the ER steps.

Victoria's grandmother helped the nurses to tenderly wipe the baby's damaged skin. I could hear murmured words: "Sweet honey, you'll be okay, let us wash you up." Through the glass ER doors, I caught sight of the shaken rookie police officer lighting his own cigarette, then the older man's. I was, for once, happy to see people smoking, for the comfort it could give. They sat close together, speaking a little and quietly, out in the darkened ambulance bay.

Finally, the police radio gave us a glimpse of the rest of the picture. Dad was incarcerated, and Mom was working her trade, under brutal circumstances, in the street. How could I condemn them, when I knew only a fragment of this horror story? How could I fix or save anyone, when clearly even God could not or had not? I could only attempt to ease the survivors and the horrified witnesses in the best way I knew how, and despite my inexperience.

I tried my best. I spoke reassuringly and kindly to the baby, the grandparents, staff, cops and paramedics, despite my fears that the baby might not make it and my inner disquiet at providing what I knew was a novice's care—earnest, but likely incomplete. I don't know why, but as I was trying to calculate antibiotic doses and IV fluid strengths and flow rates, seemingly everyone wanted to talk to "the doc." Their emotions were buffeting me, and my own heart was breaking, yet I had to maintain my composure and step up to the plate as the "doc in charge."

After my thirty-six-hour call was over, I picked up my two young daughters from daycare. I marveled at their well-fed forms and unburdened expressions. I saw their precious lives with luminous clarity, having just been shown, firsthand, how bad things could get. Despite my soiled scrubs and fatigue, we drove to the park and played on the swings for a rare, stolen half-hour before having to be home to make dinner with Daddy. My girls laughed, and I cried tears that I tried to hide—all the while thanking the powers that be that my own family was whole.

About the author: *Paula Lyons is a graduate of Emory University School of Medicine practicing family medicine just outside Baltimore, Maryland. Some of her other writings have appeared in* The Pharos *and* The Journal of Family Practice.

Late Again

Paul Gross
9/18/2009

One thing I love deeply about being a family doctor is that I get to take care of people—body and soul. A patient comes into my exam room with a litany of physical symptoms ("My shoulder...my knee...my stomach...so tired...this nausea...") and then, in response to a questioning look, suddenly bursts into tears.

It's all mine to deal with. The shoulder. The stomach. The tears. I get to gather the pieces and see if we can't put this broken person back together again.

What a privilege.

And yet the joy of primary care is also its curse. With each patient, I have to keep track of everything—the trivial and life-threatening, the physical and mental, the acute, the chronic and the preventive. And try as I might, I simply don't have enough time.

On paper, my office schedule looks simple: I see one patient every fifteen minutes beginning at 8:30 am. If I stick to my timetable, I can wrap up my twelfth patient by 11:30, finish up any leftover paperwork and enjoy an hour's lunch before starting again at 1:00.

Ha.

The reality is that I'm never done by 11:30. In fact, my colleagues and I are often still seeing our morning patients at 1:00, when our afternoon session is supposed to begin.

Lunch hour? Wouldn't it be nice.

And I have it easy. One hears of offices scheduling patients every ten minutes—*every ten minutes!*—and doctors "seeing" fifty patients a day.

Doctors talk of running on a hamster wheel. Patients complain that their doctors seem distracted, don't take the time to listen, and run late—as I routinely do.

Am I a bad doctor—disorganized and inefficient?

Or am I doomed to fall short as I bump up against powerful economic forces—the "do-more-with-less" pressures that make medical administrators everywhere create schedules like mine, designed to bring in enough money to keep health centers afloat but which end up hustling me and my patients along at an impossible pace.

As a nation, we are now trying to fix our foundering healthcare system. Before we set new rules in place, shouldn't we first ask this basic question: How much time is actually required to see a patient?

Looking for an answer, I decide to record the events and actions of a recent office visit.

Today I'm seeing Minerva Santos, an extremely nice forty-nine-year-old woman with diabetes and hypertension. Mrs. Santos is a great patient—she takes her medicines, shows up for appointments and is agreeable and uncomplaining. Compared with many other patients who are frail, in chronic pain, depressed, argumentative or uninsured, she's easy to care for.

So how long should a visit with Mrs. Santos take? Let's see.

At 8:30 this morning she walks in, placid and neatly attired, with short reddish-brown hair.

After a smile and a handshake, I tell Mrs. Santos that I'd like to review her labs and check her blood pressure. "Is there anything *you'd* like to talk about?" I ask.

"I've got a cough that's really bothering me," she says.

"Tell me about that." I add *cough* to my internal agenda. She describes a recent upper respiratory infection that flared briefly into a fever and now has her sniffling and hacking.

"Why don't I take a look in a minute?" I say.

"And I need all my prescriptions renewed," she adds. *Prescriptions*, I echo to myself.

We peer together at the computer screen. Mrs. Santos's measure of long-term diabetes control—her HbA1c—is elevated at 8.4. "We'd like to see it below seven," I tell her, "to reduce the risk of complications from your diabetes." Meanwhile, I'm wondering why her control isn't perfect.

Mrs. Santos checks her blood sugars at home; she tells me that her evening sugars are above 200 (normal is 100). Asked how she takes her diabetes medications, she says, "After eating, just like my last doctor told me to." This is odd, as they're supposed to be taken before or with meals.

We move to the examining table. I double-check her blood pressure: It's 160/100. Our goal is 130/80. Her throat, neck and lungs are unremarkable.

"Looks like a bad cold," I say. "Would you like some cough medicine?"

"Fine," she says.

She fumbles in her bag and removes seven pill bottles, a modest number for someone with her ailments. I line them up, unscrew the tops and point to the diabetes pills. Could she take them *with* dinner rather than afterwards? And how would she feel about increasing one medication's dose?

"Okay," she says.

I share my concern about her blood pressure. "It looks like you really do need a fourth blood-pressure medication. How about if I give you a new one? You'll take it once a day—with your other blood-pressure pills."

"All right," she says.

I spend several minutes printing out all of Mrs. Santos' prescriptions—four for hypertension, three for diabetes, one aspirin and one for cough. Acutely aware that I've added one new pill, changed the strength of another and altered the timing of two others—a recipe for confusion—I spend a few minutes going over all this with her.

Scanning her chart, I also notice that she needs a tetanus shot, so I order one.

Mrs. Santos leaves the exam room with a request to make an appointment for one month from now. Feeling a pang of remorse that I neglected to inquire about her family, I look at the time: 9:03. This "simple" visit has taken thirty-three minutes. And it will take more time to complete my note.

So what did I do wrong?

Well, maybe nothing—and I did accomplish quite a few things. I

- evaluated and treated Mrs. Santos' cough
- explained her lab results to her
- counseled her about the importance of diabetes and blood-pressure control
- evaluated her blood-sugar monitoring and clarified her pill regimen
- adjusted the dosage of her diabetes medications
- checked her blood pressure and prescribed a new medication
- ordered a tetanus shot and
- arranged for a follow-up visit

In addition, I also

- elicited her concerns
- assessed her understanding of our plan and
- deepened our connection

In some ways, I did a great job. But now my stomach's churning because I'm twenty minutes behind schedule. A crabby seventy-eight-year-old woman with congestive heart failure, diabetes and chronic pain is next. Can I hope to see her in fifteen minutes?

I don't think so.

Why not schedule longer visits? My health center could do that, but we'd lose money and have to fire staff and turn patients away. As it is, we already struggle to meet the needs of our vibrant, diverse Bronx community.

When I look at the big picture, I realize that I'm racing the clock partly because there aren't enough primary-care providers around. Medical students, who graduate on average more than $150,000 in debt, gravitate toward specialties that pay them more—or stress them less. In other words, they become just about any other kind of doctor.

This past year fewer than one in ten students graduating from U.S. medical schools chose residencies designed to train them in primary care. This is topsy-turvy, especially when you consider that countries with robust systems of primary care reward their citizens with better health outcomes—at lower cost—than ours does.

As our experts, policymakers and legislators take aim at our healthcare system, my plea is this: Make primary care a priority. Train more clinicians to do this critical work. Give every patient easy access to high-caliber primary care. And please...

Give me the time I need to see Mrs. Santos.

About the author: Paul Gross is editor-in-chief of Pulse—voices from the heart of medicine.

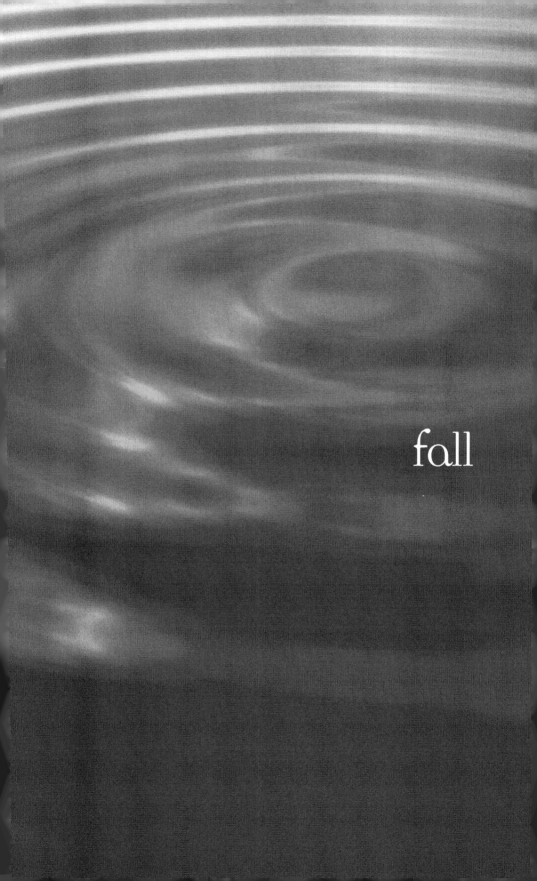

fall

first cadaver

Shanna Germain
9/25/2009

He presses the Sawzall to
her chest, slices skin to bone.
This unzipping of skin does
not stop our breaths—we're used to

invasion of the body,
the way his fingers pinch
into her pockets as though
for a cloth or a quarter.

Grasping bone ends, he spreads
her pinkish ribs, not breaking
a sweat, to find what he's come
for: such a small thing, really,

he plucks it easily.
Fingers bloodied, he holds out
the heart to us: take it, see,
it is no bigger than your fist.

About the poet: *Shanna Germain claims the titles of writer, editor, leximaven, vorpal blonde and Schrödinger's Brat. Her work has appeared in hundreds of publications, including* Absinthe Literary Review, American Journal of Nursing, Best American Erotica, McSweeney's *and* Salon. *See more of her work at* www.shannagermain.com.

About the poem: *"First Cadaver' is actually one of two poems that bookend my years of working on the ambulance. In this poem, I was trying to explore the discovery of the body, in triplicate: as it relates to our own living experiences inside our own bodies, to the dead bodies that we were seeing as part of our paramedic training, and to the living bodies of our patients."*

steep sledding

Jonathan Han
10/2/2009

"Don't worry," my doctor said.

I barely heard what he was saying; lying there in the hospital bed, I was caught up in contemplating the diagnostic procedure I was scheduled to have the next morning.

"With these anesthetics," he continued, "you won't feel or remember a thing after it's over."

"Okay," I answered weakly, signing the consent form with unaccustomed legibility. But could I really forget the emotional trauma of these past twelve hours?

I'm a physician, and blessedly accustomed to standing on the other side of the health-and-illness divide. But after four days of crampy abdominal pain, my self-diagnosed "gastroenteritis" had horribly morphed into a "rule out carcinoma" directive. Now I faced another twelve hours of waiting—reviewing the possibilities, expecting the worst—until my procedure could be performed. Could I stop silently reviewing my CAT scan findings (that suspicious abdominal mass) and numb my feelings of anguish and anticipatory grief?

"Do you want a sleeping pill for tonight?" asked my doctor.

"I don't know," I stammered.

"It may help you sleep," he pressed.

"Okay," I said, grasping at the chance to escape this nightmare. Inwardly, though, I craved normal sleep complete with dreams, not anesthesia's timeless, dreamless fugue state.

A brief visit from my wife and two young children helped me feel almost normal again. My wife Marilyn, as supportive and hopeful as usual, told me that she still thought my symptoms could be the result of an infection. "Let's see what the test shows first, and we'll move on from there."

However, it wasn't long before I returned to worrying that our future together might be cut terribly short.

Fortunately, my children distracted themselves, and me, by pointing out the vagaries of hospital-bed controls.

"Dad, wouldn't it be great to have a bed that moved like this at home?" asked my son Davey as the foot of the hospital bed whirred slowly up and down.

The highlight, for me, was watching my seven-year-old daughter Grace skipping down the hospital hallway as she headed for the elevators to leave. Her carefree skipping was a precious invitation to forget my anxiety and enjoy the moment, and I did.

After they left, I endured two hours of cable-TV cooking shows until the nurse finally brought in my benzodiazepine nightcap.

"This will never work," I thought, closing my eyes and tugging my stiff white sheets out of their hospital corners.

But I was wrong.

Half an hour later, it seemed, I found myself standing in my front yard in midwinter, staring down the small slope that led to the street. Grace, clad in snowsuit and red-striped stocking ski cap, smiled broadly at me as she mounted a sled.

"Don't worry," she told me. "It'll be all right."

Then she was off, squealing with delight as the snow swirled behind her, and picking up speed as the hill somehow grew steeper and longer. She was heading for the street—and straight for our neighbor's house.

"Wait, stop!" I screamed. I ran down the hill, trying to keep her from getting hit by a car or plowing head-first into our neighbor's front porch.

Instead, Grace accelerated, laughing all the way to the bottom. She hit a bump and started flying through the air.

I stood staring in disbelief and horror as she gained altitude, climbing impossibly high up over my neighbor's house and ancient hemlock tree, then dropping down and disappearing into their backyard, her striped ski cap a tiny flame flickering goodbye.

In a panic, I dashed behind the neighbor's house and found Grace.

She was making a snow angel. Snowflakes glistening on her nose, she cheerfully greeted me.

"That was fun! Let's do it again!"

"Okay," I said with relief.

Just then, the nurse tugged at my hospital gown.

"Wake up, it's time for your morning medications. They'll be taking you down for your procedure in a few minutes."

I looked around the hospital room. My IV was still running, the nurses' call button was still at my side, and the institutional green walls still needed a fresh coat of paint; but everything looked different somehow.

The same was true for me. I was still facing the same uncertainties and fears, but they didn't feel so terrible now. Something had shifted inside.

"All right," I replied. "I'm ready."

About the author: Family physician Jonathan Han is medical director of New Kensington Family Health Center at University of Pittsburg Medical Center (UPMC) and a faculty member at UPMC St. Margaret Family Practice Residency Program. "I started writing about medicine after attending an inspiring

Society of Teachers of Family Medicine workshop led by Paul Gross. Writing is a wonderful way to focus my attention on the things I care about, and to slow down and try to enjoy the moment. The diagnostic procedure described in my story, a colonoscopy, revealed that I had Crohn's disease—a difficult diagnosis, but one that I welcomed, given the alternative. Being a parent and a physician, I am constantly learning lessons about humility. Had my diagnosis indeed been cancer, I hope I would have had the strength and grace to have written this story, because the lesson that Grace taught me in the dream—that I would get through the challenge ahead, no matter what—still remains."

second-guessed

Andrea Gordon
10/9/2009

It was a good night, but it's been a brutal morning.

As a family doctor who does obstetrics, I generally enjoy my time with laboring patients. When I arrived on the maternity floor last night to start my call, things looked pleasantly uneventful. Several patients were in labor. Only one wasn't progressing well: Ana, age twenty-two.

I was told that Ana had come to the floor two days earlier, leaking puddles of clear fluid but not contracting. She still wasn't contracting, even after two days on Pitocin, the drug that causes or strengthens uterine contractions.

To add to this difficulty, there was Ana's shift nurse, Barbara.

Barbara and I had a history. Another night, caring for a very annoying patient, I'd thought that Barbara had acted unprofessionally, and she'd accused me of shirking my responsibilities. We hadn't parted on the best of terms.

As the night wore on, Ana's uterus finally began to contract, but she didn't tolerate the discomfort well. She was also fearful of taking any pain medication—a perfect catch-22.

Avoiding a replay of our last collaboration, Barbara and I managed to soothe Ana and her husband, and they changed their minds about Ana's getting an epidural.

Now pain-free, Ana got a steady dose of Pitocin all night long. And I got a four-and-a-half-hour block of sleep—a luxury on OB call.

The next morning, Barbara woke me before 6:00.

"Can you check Ana?" she asked. "If she hasn't made any progress, can we turn off the 'pit' and call it a day?" By this, she meant schedule Ana for the C-section that she'd been promised if her cervix didn't dilate overnight.

Under my gloved fingers, Ana's cervix felt unchanged. The baby's head seemed asynclitic (turned to the side and not well applied to the cervix), which might explain why Ana wasn't dilating well. And I didn't feel any bulging bag of amniotic fluid, which went along with her history of leaking dramatically. The C-section looked more and more certain.

But the obstetricians on call weren't happy with this plan: They had two other C-sections already scheduled.

How sure was I that Ana's water had broken? they asked.

Ninety-plus percent, based on my exam, I said, then related my concerns about the baby's head position.

Dr. Jarvis, the obstetrician coming on for the day, decided to examine Ana herself.

Looking at Ana's fetal monitoring strip, she said, "She's not contracting!"

I explained that we'd turned off the Pitocin to give the patient a break. She pointed out, rightly, that with the epidural in place, Ana hadn't been uncomfortable.

I mentally kicked myself.

Mistake number one: Wanting to avoid a confrontation with Barbara, I'd simply agreed when she had suggested turning off the pit. Given Ana's tepid progress, I'd also believed that it wouldn't make much difference.

Reviewing the tracings that recorded Ana's progress, Dr. Jarvis said, "Her contractions haven't been adequate."

I bridled: Ana *had* been uncomfortable; Barbara and I had agreed that her contractions had felt moderate; she'd been contracting for more than twelve hours. And yet....

Mistake number two: Before turning off Ana's Pitocin, I should have given her the highest possible dose and asked to be awakened after two hours so that I could check her progress and maybe insert an intra-uterine pressure catheter to measure her contraction strength. But between wanting to minimize the number of exams (which increase the risk of infection in a woman whose sac has ruptured) and feeling that higher doses of Pitocin wouldn't help anyway, maybe I'd closed that door too soon. Or maybe I just didn't want to fight with Barbara about it.

Or maybe, if I was to be brutally honest with myself, I just wanted to sleep.

Dr. Jarvis checked Ana. "I feel a bag. She's not ruptured. Hook, please."

I handed her an amniotomy hook. Clear fluid came running out.

To complete my humiliation, Dr. Jarvis said, "And she's not asynclitic; she's left occiput anterior"—a perfectly normal position for the baby's head.

Mistakes three and four. Missed the sac. Got the head position wrong.

Part of being a family doctor who does obstetrics is being second-guessed by the specialists—the ob-gyns whom you consult when you have concerns or need a surgical intervention. Often your judgment is found wanting.

This can be tormenting, because in obstetrics, as in all of medicine, you can do the right thing and have a bad outcome. Or you can do the wrong thing and have everything turn out well. Also, the lack of scientific evidence for many protocols used in childbirth, and the potential for catastrophic outcomes, makes everyone's emotions run high. In this high-stakes situation, specialists tend to support their opinions with a nonscientific phrase: "In my experience." It's unanswerable because, as the specialists, they do have the most experience.

I walked into the staff room to find my morning replacement there with some nurses. When I described what had happened, they told me not to take it personally. Dr. Jarvis was known for her brusqueness, and it had been reasonable for me to turn off the Pitocin.

Mulling it all over in the light of day, I'd like to believe that they were right—but I feel at least partially culpable. And as the night's events go round and round in my head, there's what I come up with:

- I tried to help Ana deliver vaginally, but because I was pessimistic about her chances, I didn't push hard to give her every chance.

- We minimized the number of exams to lower the risk of infection.

- I didn't want to fight with Barbara.

- When Barbara expressed discomfort with giving Ana a high dose of Pitocin, I didn't think it would make a difference, so I went along.

- I was asleep at 2 am and happy to remain so, knowing that the following evening I'd be the sole caregiver for my very active toddler.

- Finally, when I examined Ana's cervix at 6 am, maybe I didn't check as thoroughly as I should have.

It's possible that my exam isn't as proficient as I'd like to think. (One study shows that obstetricians, using vaginal exams, get the baby's position right just 50 percent of the time—so maybe no one is all that good.) But it's just as possible that something changed during the two hours between my exam and Dr. Jarvis's. Maybe the baby's head shifted and the amniotic bag became more apparent.

There's no way to know.

Perhaps I'd feel some vindication if Ana needed a C-section after all, but the last I heard, she was contracting well and headed for a vaginal delivery.

All that I can do is to ask what I might have done better—then try and do it. Next time, which will be next week, I want to stay more aware of my potential biases and try to sidestep or blast through them. Dr. Jarvis may have been arrogant, but that doesn't let me off the hook.

So it may have been a good night, but it's been a hell of a morning.

―――――――――――

About the author: *Andrea Gordon is on the faculty of the Tufts Family Medicine Residency Program at Cambridge Health Alliance in Malden, Massachusetts. "Although I wrote poetry in high school, I had stopped until my advisor in residency told me, 'You should write poetry.' That was enough to start me writing again. I feel privileged to be invited into people's lives and to hear their stories. I try to make time to reflect when not distracted by my five-year-old-son, brilliant husband and two needy cats. Oh, and work!"*

Reading Entrails

Kenneth P. Gurney
10/16/2009

Sugar poisons
ruin your blood,
runs your legs
while you sleep,
revs your irregular
heart beat.

Maple sap, tree ripened
orange, dark chocolate,
honey dripping
from the comb
are not viable substitutes;
only abstinence
and the eleven day
skin crawl withdrawal.

Or an asymmetrical death:
one part at a time,
organ by organ,
memory fog,
the surgeons gnawing
like rats
at the leper's limbs.

About the poet: *Kenneth P. Gurney lives in Albuquerque, NM, with his beloved Dianne. He edits* Adobe Walls, *an anthology of works by New Mexico poets. His latest book is* This is not Black & White. *To learn more, visit* www.kpgurney. me/poet/Welcome.html.

About the poem: *"A few people I know are/were in denial about their adult-onset diabetes. So I wrote and performed this piece a couple of times in public in the hope of jarring them into taking care of themselves. One of these people did go through sugar-withdrawal heebie-jeebies for what he said seemed like forever but was really about ten days. The title comes from the ancient augury practice of reading the entrails of a sacrificed animal to predict the future; the twist here is that it's the diabetic's insides that do the prognostication."*

one more child left behind

Brian T. Maurer
10/23/12

Making the diagnosis might be straightforward, but sometimes getting adequate medical care poses a more formidable challenge.

It was the end of an exhausting afternoon in our busy pediatric practice in Enfield, Connecticut. I had just finished seeing what I thought was the last patient of the day, only to find yet another chart resting in the wall rack, a silent signal that one more patient waited behind an adjacent closed door.

His name was Aaron. Six years old, he sat on the exam table cradling his left arm in his lap. The most striking thing about the arm was the large bluish bulge on the side of his elbow. His mother stood by his side; his grandmother sat in the corner chair.

"What happened?" I asked.

"Another kid pushed him off a table at school. He won't move his arm."

I took a step closer. "Let's have a look."

Gently, I palpated the borders of the blue bulge. Aaron winced in pain. I felt his wrist to check the circulation to his hand. "Squeeze my fingers," I said. He tried and winced again.

"It's likely broken," I explained. "At this hour all the x-ray facilities in town are closed. Your best bet is to take him to the emergency room," I continued, wrapping Aaron's arm in a sling.

"When you get to the hospital, they'll take a special picture of your arm," I told him. "Give them a big grin so it comes out well, okay?"

Aaron's grandmother flashed a faint smile as they walked out.

The next morning Aaron's mother phoned the office to tell me that, although the x-ray showed a fracture of the elbow, no "bone doctor" had come to the hospital to treat the break. Instead, she was given the names of some local orthopedic surgeons, with instructions to arrange an appointment with one of them that morning. But none of the surgeons would give her an appointment, so she wanted advice about what to do.

When I flipped through Aaron's chart, I saw why none of the local orthopedists would see him. It was all too clear: Aaron's health insurance coverage was through an underfunded state-sponsored Medicaid plan.

I telephoned the client services department of Aaron's health plan. A cordial representative proceeded to give me the names of several participating orthopedic doctors in the area.

"Hold on," I interrupted her when I heard the first name. "The mother already called that practice and was told they were no longer participating."

"Sometimes that happens," the representative told me. "The doctor opts out, but doesn't inform us directly, so we still have the name on our list." She gave me three other names and telephone numbers. "Call me if you're still having a problem," she said cheerfully. "Have a nice day."

Feeling frustrated and irritable, I delegated the task of locating a participating provider to Laura, one of our medical assistants. "When you find someone, schedule the appointment and call the mother to let her know," I told her, then turned my attention to my morning patients.

I returned from lunch to find Laura still on the phone. "None of the practices you gave me would accept this kid's insurance," she said. "I called client services again and got six more names. Each office was happy to schedule an appointment until I told them the insurance carrier. I can't believe that no one will see a six-year-old boy with a broken arm!"

"We'll demand an out-of-network pre-authorization for care and send him to Children's Hospital in Hartford," I said, gritting my teeth. "I'd rather he be seen by a pediatric orthopedic specialist anyway." And I knew that Children's Hospital was just a half-hour drive away.

Somehow Laura got the pre-authorization approved and called Children's. I heard the phone slam down, then her footsteps resounded in the hallway.

"This is absolutely crazy!" she cried. "They won't see him, even with a pre-authorization! Now what?"

I rubbed my forehead as though it were Aladdin's lamp. At this point I needed a magic genie. I was running out of options.

"Why not try the orthopedic clinic at University Hospital?" our office manager suggested. I knew that only adult orthopedic surgeons worked there—and that it was further away.

"It's a long shot, but—call them," I said, conscious of the tightness in my neck.

A few minutes later, Laura shouted, "University Hospital will see him!" She was ecstatic. "They take his insurance!"

My jaw dropped. "Wow. Great! So now all we have to do is tell this mother she has to drive an hour to have her child attended by a participating doctor."

I glanced at the clock. All told, we had placed eighteen phone calls over four hours to get one child the care he needed. When he was finally attended at University Hospital, twenty-four hours had elapsed since the time of his injury.

When this incident occurred, in 2003, 43 million Americans had no health insurance. Since then, the number of uninsured has grown to 47 million. With widespread unemployment generated by our current economic crisis, new members are added to these ranks daily. As a nation, we are now wrestling with the question of how to give all Americans adequate health insurance coverage.

The irony here is that Aaron *had* insurance. His story reminds us that threadbare health coverage is no great help or solace in time of real need.

Unfortunately, his experience is not uncommon in a system that unofficially rations care and delays appropriate treatment.

As one of the world's wealthiest nations, we have the resources to make sure that all of our citizens have timely access to affordable, high-quality health care. We should see that they get it.

Otherwise, patients like Aaron will continue to slip through the cracks— one child at a time.

(A previous version of this piece appeared in the online journal Dermanities *and was subsequently published in* Patients Are a Virtue: Clinical Tales in the Art of Medicine.*)*

About the author: *Brian T. Maurer has practiced pediatric medicine as a physician assistant for the past three decades. As a clinician, he has always gravitated toward the humane aspect of patient care—what he calls the soul of medicine. Over the past decade, Brian has explored the illness narrative as a tool to enhance the education of medical students and to cultivate an appreciation for the delivery of humane medical care. To date he has published two collections of stories,* Patients Are a Virtue *and* Village Voices. *He can also be found at his blog,* briantmaurer.wordpress.com.

The Resilient Heart

Paula Lyons
10/30/2009

He was applying for a job on a refuse truck working for the City. This is a very good job for someone whose hiring prospects are otherwise limited. Excellent benefits, all state and federal holidays off, health insurance for oneself and one's family, physical exercise in the fresh air. (All right, this was Camden, New Jersey, so exercise in *some* kind of air.) And one more plus: If the team is efficient and hardworking and get through their rounds by 11:30 am or noon, they can take the rest of the day off, yet get paid as if they'd worked the whole 5 am-to-1 pm shift.

I was the doctor doing his pre-placement physical exam—designed to determine if the potential employee has medical conditions or takes medicines (or recreational drugs) that might interfere with the employee "performing essential job functions in a safe, regular, and reliable fashion."

He was twenty-five, slender but muscular, and very excited about the prospect of this job. He was polite and engaging. He surely was capable of lifting cans into the "load-packer" and running beside, or hanging onto the side of, the trash truck as it went on its rounds cleaning up the City.

I took a basic medical and social history. No medicines, a nonsmoker, no prior work injuries. All good news. Never graduated high school: "I ain't no scholar, that's for sure."

Some marijuana use in the past, but "I don't do that shit no more, doc, I got a family to take care of."

"Have you ever had to be in the hospital overnight, besides being born?"

"Well, yeah, doc—I got a surgery. I got stabbed in the aorta."

He proudly opened the flowered cotton gown to display a raised, thick, vertical scar that bisected his chest between his impressive pecs. Just below, I saw a smaller, horizontal scar—surely the entry point of the assailant's knife.

I had believed my patient's declaration even before I saw the scars, knowing from our previous conversation that the word "aorta" was unlikely to be part of his everyday vocabulary. Clearly, he'd been schooled in essential anatomy during his stay at Shock Trauma (or, as the Trauma Center was locally referred to by docs and layfolk alike, "Shock-a-Rama").

Despite this incontrovertible visible evidence, I was amazed: The aorta is the largest artery in the body, and direct trauma to it is almost invariably fatal.

I goggled.

"Yup," he said, nodding at my thunderstruck expression. "Got me right below my breastbone, and even nicked my heart."

"Oh my God!" I sputtered. "What happened? Who stabbed you?"

"Well," he admitted with a wry grin, "It was my baby-mama. We was at a wedding, and we was drinkin', and we got to arguing, and she stabbed me. The paramedics said if I hadn't been drunk, I'da been dead."

What a sobering tale. A wedding disrupted by a crime of passion. A drunken altercation that nearly led to a young man's death. At least one child's life forever altered by this terrible happening: Mother attempts to murder Father. I was appalled, but did my best to conceal it.

I couldn't control my curiosity, though. Fearing the answer, but feeling compelled, I asked, "Where...where is she now?"

"Oh," he replied casually, "She home with the children. Now we has four. Oldest is seven, youngest is almost two. I didn't press no charges, and she didn't have no record, and we carried it off, with the state defender helpin', as a sorta 'tragic accident.' Now I is quite careful not to look at other women, and we has no problems."

He smiled, his excellent teeth gleaming. His optimism was infectious.

I finished his exam, my head in a whirl, and reported to the City that this man was well-equipped to be employed.

Shaking my hand vigorously, he thanked me again and again. Yet I had done nothing extraordinary. I had just told the simple truth—this man was clearly capable of doing the job to which he aspired.

"I can't wait to tell Maria and the kids; they is gonna be so glad."

In the days that followed, I couldn't help but wonder about my patient's life. Having little data with which to develop an accurate picture, I was left with questions that surely reflected my own view of the world rather than his.

I've tried to envision this happy-go-lucky, plucky survivor in his own world. He will now have a steady job—which will, among other things, pay for his family's medical care. When he comes home some weeks hence smelling of trash truck, will he toss his toddler gently into the air and listen happily to the excited squeals that mean "Daddy is home"? At night, when he sleeps, will his woman trace the scars on his chest with tentative fingers and reflect?

My patient and his family life are foreign to me, yet they have intersected mine via a thirty-minute pre-placement assessment. I want, I need, I hope to understand. I crave to know the secret of my patient's resilient heart—to fathom the bedrock truths that allow him to smile, to hope, to maintain his family intact.

My patient's world view—his truths—*must* possess awesome power and healing force. Witness the fact that this man's wounds (the devastating physical ones and the no less complicated emotional ones) have been overcome, and that he remains a joyous, hopeful soul who exults in his connection with his woman and children. The result? Six people (some might call them disadvantaged) are bound by history, circumstance, routine and, clearly, love. They have endured and survived as a cohesive unit. Together, as a family, they have endured and transcended a most shocking instance of violence.

When I feel depleted, when my husband and I quarrel or one of the girls brings home a less than ideal report from school, I try, before reacting, to think about my Man of the Resilient Heart. How important are our relatively small problems compared to his past and present challenges? I aspire to attain his level of commitment to family and his incredibly learned acceptance of the imperfect in the people he so dearly loves.

About the author: *Paula Lyons is a native of New Jersey who graduated from Emory University School of Medicine. She now practices family medicine just outside of Baltimore, MD. Some of her other writings have appeared in* The Pharos *and* The Journal of Family Practice.

My Evidence

Cortney Davis
11/5/2009

When I saw dust settling,
the road black and gritty,

and noticed the air
shimmering as it lowered closer to the earth

like a soft blanket suffocating
the damp September

mornings that had morphed seamlessly
into November's

crowded table
of berries, sweets, and yellow corn,

just before the hospital
phoned to say that Mother had called my name,

familiar syllables
caught in her throat,

I'd already detected her leaving
in my own body

and so while she paused
at the end of her journey,

which was also the beginning,
I rushed to her,

hurrying
as I'd never hurried before.

About the poet: Cortney Davis is a nurse practitioner, poet and essayist. "I've been writing since my childhood, encouraged by my mother who loved poetry, and my father, a writer himself, who would type up the first few sentences of a story and ask me to finish it. I've never stopped writing since." Cortney's latest book is The Heart's Truth: Essays on the Art of Nursing, *winner of an Independent Publisher Book Awards Silver Medal in Nonfiction and an American Journal of Nursing Book of the Year Award. Other publications are listed on her Web site,* www.cortneydavis.com.

About the poem: "The poem 'My Evidence' began as a workshop exercise—write a poem in which you use the words 'dust,' 'blanket' and so on. But then, somewhere in the middle, the memory of my mother's death came into the poem, totally unexpectedly. At that point I abandoned the 'exercise' and let the poem go where it would."

Help me

Jennifer Reckrey
11/13/2009

Editor's Note: Jennifer Reckrey kept a weekly journal of her experiences during her intern year.

Week 13

I had a few free minutes at the end of my clinic session this past Thursday morning, so I took over a walk-in patient from an overbooked colleague.

The patient was a large, muscular Salvadoran man in his early forties who had long-standing hypertension. He said that for the past three months, he'd been feeling tired and didn't have the energy to take his daily medications. Just a few months back, he'd finished a five-year prison sentence for armed robbery. Now he was living temporarily with his twenty-year-old daughter and her boyfriend, but he told me that he couldn't seem to get his feet back on the ground. Though he made a little money here and there as a freelance mechanic, he couldn't get steady work: No one wanted to employ a felon, and the job-placement program couldn't help him because of his mental illness.

"What mental illness?" I asked.

Looking more at the wall than at me, he described voices that he'd heard ever since he was a boy. Though the voices had started out as benign whispers, they'd eventually become angry and mean. They regularly told him to kill himself, and in the past he had tried. Sometimes they faded a bit, but in the last few months they'd been getting louder and more directive by the day. They told him not to take his pills. They told him that people on the street were out to get him and couldn't be trusted. They told him to jump in front of oncoming subway trains. And it was getting harder to ignore them, harder to say no.

He looked right at me: "But I don't want to die."

He was so earnest and insightful, yet also so needy and overwhelmed. Feeling instant empathy, I assured him that it was no wonder that he couldn't take his medications or find a job. And I promised to do what I could to help him get the voices under control.

But what? The routine protocol for patients suffering from command auditory hallucinations instructing suicide is immediate evaluation in a psychiatric ER. But he had a car-repair job lined up in Brooklyn that afternoon and was counting on the income to buy groceries. He'd survived with these voices for twenty years, and I didn't think it was necessary to get the police involved to force him to go to the ER right then. But he did need to get there soon. It was unlikely that he would be admitted to the hospital, but the ER was required by law to make sure that he had a follow-up appointment with a mental health worker within five days. And this was essential. A psych referral for a Medicaid patient in the Bronx can take weeks. Or more.

So with the help of the clinic social worker and my supervising physician, we made a plan. That afternoon he would do his job in Brooklyn and immediately afterward would bring my handwritten referral letter to the psychiatric ER so he could be evaluated.

The next day, both the social worker and I checked the hospital computer system: He hadn't gone to the ER. I called him, and he told me that he was still busy in Brooklyn but was feeling okay. He said he appreciated my call and would go to the ER soon. Three days later he hadn't gone to the hospital, and neither the social worker nor I could reach him by phone. She decided that we needed to call a community-based suicide intervention team to visit his last listed address and assess him again. He wasn't there. They said they will keep trying.

Since then, I've called him twice, and there's been no answer. I think of him often—of the resilience it takes to grow into an articulate and thoughtful man despite hearing a constant, disembodied voice telling you that you are worthless. And I find myself checking my workplace voicemail more often than usual, even when I'm not in clinic, hoping to hear that he's all right.

Week 18

I stopped by the clinic social worker's basement office this week to see if she had heard from the suicidal, hallucinating patient we'd seen a few weeks back. She hadn't. The suicide intervention team had attempted several times to evaluate him at home, but he'd never been there. They'd spoken to his adult daughter, who'd told them he was in Brooklyn and doing fine. And so they had "closed the file."

I turned to leave, but the social worker stopped me. Turning from her desk, she asked softly, "Did you learn anything from this case?"

This is what she wanted to hear me say: When someone hears voices commanding him to kill himself, there is no room for negotiation. An immediate professional evaluation is both clinically and legally necessary to avoid situations like the one we were in right now.

But I couldn't bring myself to say it.

I have learned so much over these last months. When lab tests revealed that my patient's vague abdominal pain was actually severe pancreatitis, I learned to take every complaint seriously. When my uninsured patient stopped taking her seizure medication because it wasn't covered at her sliding-scale pharmacy, I learned that having one detail out of place can topple a whole treatment plan. But this was different. And much more difficult.

I hate that there are so few social services available to help poor people maintain their health, and that getting a life started again after incarceration is an almost insurmountable task. I hate that mental health care is so isolated from the rest of medicine, that even individuals who want help can lose months of their lives waiting for the referral to come through.

I want to swoop in and guide my patient through this complicated system. I also want to respect his decisions and honor the instinct for survival that has brought him this far. And I don't know how to reconcile these two desires.

I still have so much more to learn.

About the author: Jennifer Reckrey MD *wrote this when she was a family-medicine resident in New York City. "I started writing these reflections to keep in touch with friends and family, but they soon became a valuable way for me to understand my own developing practice of medicine."*

Maman

Paul Gross
11/20/2009

At a recent religious service I attended with Maman, my eighty-seven-year-old mother, I watched her fumbling attempts to find hymn number 123, "Spirit of Life," in her hymnal. I held my book up, opened to the appropriate page, so that we both could sing from it.

She glanced up momentarily, tightened her lips, hunched forward and resumed turning pages, finally arriving at the song as the congregation was singing the second verse, which she needed help finding—what with her poor vision and the swirl of notes and words on the page.

As this ritual repeated itself, hymn after hymn, it occurred to me how much cozier it would be if my mother and I could share the same hymnal.

It also struck to me how unlike Maman that would be. Her need to do things independently—and the improbability of Maman reciting from someone else's page—capture in a nutshell the difficulties we've experienced with her aging process.

Maman was born in Belgium in 1922. She lived through the Nazi occupation before coming to the U.S. Of her five siblings, only one sister remains.

My father died seven years ago after a lengthy battle with prostate cancer. His death left Maman alone, isolated and without her prime purpose in life—caring for, cajoling and trying to exert her will over my dad. He played the immovable object to her irresistible force. Without another person upon whom to focus her indomitable spirit, she seemed to lose energy. And showed increasing signs of forgetfulness.

A couple of years later, Maman had an explosive falling out with her closest friend in the world, her remaining sister, in a Walmart in Florida. They've rarely spoken since.

She started getting lost en route to our house. Eventually, after a traffic accident, she mercifully gave up driving—without ever acknowledging a reason.

As she started to slide, we pleaded with her to plan ahead. "I'll cross that bridge when I get to it," she said. Then, one day, there she was, on the bridge, swaying above the chasm.

She lost her wallet on a bus, but couldn't remember what bus it was, why she was on it, or even that she'd been on a bus—and then lost the piece of paper with the phone number of the good Samaritan who'd found her wallet.

While out walking, she fell on the sidewalk and broke her nose.

She'd call my brother Eric—an internist with a large geriatric practice—weeping. "I'm lonely." The next day she'd insist that she wasn't lonely at all, that she couldn't remember calling him and that she was never bored and "happy as an angel."

Her circle of acquaintances shrank: a neighbor who'd occasionally stop by. Her building doormen. And, most critically, Sandy—"Poochi!"—an outgoing miniature Chihuahua that Eric gave her.

Through all this she responded with outbursts to any attempts at discussion.

"I'm not lonely! You think I'm crazy! You want to lock me away! If you do, I'll throw myself from the roof!"

On my family's weekly visits, I'd survey her refrigerator.

"There's no food here," I'd say.

"That's all right," she'd answer. "I can go out any time I want."

"What did you have for lunch?" I'd ask.

"Oh, I don't know," she'd answer dismissively.

The irony—two physicians with a mother who was living alone, poorly nourished, with no memory to speak of (who knew if she was taking her pills?) and at high risk of falling—was not lost on Eric and me. And yet we wavered in the face of her fierce will, electing to wait until some disaster—a broken hip, a stroke, an accident crossing the street—suddenly and irrevocably changed the equation.

But something else happened. The tectonic plates continued to shift, further eroding her memory and her fight.

During a recent month-long stay with Eric upstate, he tried to interest her in an assisted-care facility, with predictable results. But then, eyeing her diminishing faculties, he also refused to take her home.

And we held our breaths.

The furious assault she might have launched a year earlier never happened. It was as if her army's tanks had rusted, the soldiers had gotten tired and, most critically, the generals were too distracted to care that there was a war on.

Maman is now staying with us for the month of November. In December she'll return to Eric's house. She is sleeping on our ground-floor living-room sofa, having tumbled down our stairs a year ago. "But I never fall," she says, when we discuss the stairs with her.

Our daughters' former caregiver Marie is now back, looking after Maman several hours a day. Even as they go out for walks or sit on the couch watching a Fred Astaire-Ginger Rogers movie, Maman thinks Marie is only here to tidy up the house.

Much of the time she's typically hyper-cheerful, laughing at Sandy's antics ("Come on, Poochi!"), her blue eyes bright and a little blank, her blonde hair now straw-like. She wears the same clothes for days on end. When she smelled of pee one day, and I suggested that perhaps Marie could help her with a bath, she glared at me. Later that day, with a tight grip on the railing, she inched up the stairs—alone and muttering—to bathe.

In the evening she becomes sad and disoriented. I've come upon her sobbing.

"I'm lonely," she says. "I wish I could go to sleep and not wake up. I'll take Sandy with me."

At night, I find her emptying out the wrong kitchen cabinet—peanut butter and jam jars on the counter—in a futile search for tea.

"Do you find that you get a little confused in the evening, or that it's harder to remember things?" I ask her.

"No."

As I head upstairs to bed, I hear her poking around the kitchen, removing dirty dishes from the dishwasher, "cleaning" them and putting them away in the cupboard, where we'll find them, still slippery with grease, in the morning.

"Frying pan...frying pan...frying pan..." I hear her whispering.

The ground is constantly giving way on this journey. We now find ourselves on a stable ledge. But what will the next tremor bring? Wandering? Another fall? A more furious outburst?

Given that my brother and I are doctors, it's ironic that the medical profession rarely enters into our discussions. Maybe it's because neither of us thinks that physicians have much to offer at the moment; in fact, we seem to agree that the best we can do medically is to keep Maman out of the grips of a hospital, where she would only get worse.

What ails Maman is beyond tests and medicines. Just like her last bit of retained memory—the one that says, "I don't need any help!"—that won't show up on any scan.

"I'm glad you're here," she says, hugging me one night in our living room. Then confusion flickers across her face. "You're not going home?"

"No, Maman, we're staying here tonight with you."

"Good!"

For now.

About the author: *Paul Gross is a family physician and founding editor of* Pulse—voices from the heart of medicine.

cleft

Jon Neher
11/27/2009

As Caroline was born
the doctor saw
the split
from lip to nose—
purple rimmed,
going down deep—
Deep enough
to hurt
generations.

And the imperfect doctor,
tired of wounds
tired of divisions,
saw the small
wholeness
Chose that moment
Chose tenderness
saying simply,
She is beautiful.

And the imperfect mother,
tired of pain,
held her child,
touched the tiny,
ragged face
Chose that moment
Chose acceptance
crying softly,
She is beautiful.

About the poet: *Jon Neher is clinical professor of family medicine at the University of Washington in Seattle and associate director of the Valley Medical Center Family Medicine Residency Program. He is editor-in-chief of the newsletter* Evidence-Based Practice *and a frequent contributor of essays on medical education to* Family Medicine.

About the poem: *"This poem was written to capture the layering of emotions that occurred the day I unexpectedly delivered an infant with a cleft palate. I was new to my career, and this was a novel challenge for me. Since I had no professional scripting to fall back on, and because I wanted to encourage bonding, I found myself repeatedly saying how beautiful the baby was, even as I discussed the cleft with the parents. The effect on the family was precisely what I was hoping for."*

MOM

Diane Guernsey
12/5/2009

By this time next week, my mother may be dead.

In a sense, she's been dying for a long time. This leg of her journey is the last in a decades-long trek with Parkinson's disease.

She lies there, her head small and delicate on the pillow. Her hair is a wispy white thatch; her throat muscles are rigid, as if she's lifting a huge barbell. Her breaths come slowly, with long pauses in between; she sounds nearly too tired to go on. Her brown eyes stare up, half-open, sightless.

This nursing facility is part of the stepped-care retirement center where my parents moved more than ten years ago, anticipating the day when Mom would need more help than Dad could give her. They lived in an apartment there for years, while Parkinson's slowly chilled my mom's brisk, jaunty gestures and muffled her lively, Texas-inflected conversation into an inaudible murmur. (We all knew that her deterioration was inevitable, despite the excellent care her doctors provided.) When a stroke unexpectedly felled my dad seven years ago, my mom, then eighty, chose to move into the facility's nursing wing.

About a month ago, Mom basically stopped eating. She dwindled down to eighty-five pounds on her five-foot-seven frame. That's when Dr. Greene, the facility physician, called in the hospice staff.

A hospice nurse told us the jarring news: Mom would be lucky to make it through the end of November.

My brothers and I flew in—they from the West Coast, I from New York. Now I'm back at Mom's bedside for another visit, a couple of days before Thanksgiving.

Medical science has given Mom a lot. But the Parkinson's pills are useless now, and so much of the rest is chilly and inhuman: the shiny plastic oxygen tube that snakes beneath her nostrils; the tinny whirr and sigh of the oxygen machine. For me, this machine sums it all up—the human wish to help, the imperfection of the attempt. "It's not doing much for her," admits Mom's nurse, Charlotte. To me, Charlotte's gentle voice and soft hands seem to the only truly healing things in the whole set-up.

There's only so much anyone can do, no matter how well-intentioned. The hospice people offer comforting words, but their soothing professional tones somehow remind me of artificial pancake syrup. I'm being ungrateful, I know. It's not their fault that they can't give Mom back to me.

Someone has dressed her in a pretty, lace-edged sleeveless nightgown. It doesn't hide much. Her body could be a living anatomy lesson—skeletal, graceful, each tendon sharply picked out. Her cheekbones jut out beneath her hollowed eye sockets. Her eyebrows arch in a look of elegant surprise. Her mouth gapes, gasping slightly with every breath, slower and shallower with each passing hour. When the nurses shift her in bed, I see her arms and legs, long and lean and bony as a colt's. Sadness wells inside me.

Mom was pretty, spirited and energetic. "Once a Texan, always a Texan," she'd say proudly. And she had a knack for making friends and connecting with people. "She can talk to anyone," my dad said admiringly—and since I was shy like him, I shared his wonder as Mom chatted easily with the Disneyland ticket takers or the guards at the museums to which she and Dad dragged us kids.

Mom's social smarts, curiosity and love of learning would have made her a natural teacher, social worker or journalist, but lack of money made it impossible for her to finish college—a lifelong regret. Like most women of her generation, she plowed her talents into homemaking, tracking her children's progress or misdeeds and volunteering for the PTA and the League of Women Voters.

We didn't always get on well when I was growing up. Our temperaments differed, and our rapport frayed as I entered my teens. We were hard on each other—angry and hurtful, sometimes on purpose. I remember how Mom once criticized me to near-tears while she was trimming my hair in front of the bathroom mirror. As I bit my trembling lip, she snapped scornfully, "Why don't you just *cry*?" Another time, I reduced her to wounded silence by sneering, "I'm smarter than you."

After college, I kept things cordial but safely distant, fearful of more storms and scared that, otherwise, I couldn't ever become truly independent.

Years later, well launched in my career, married and with a baby daughter, I felt a yearning for more closeness with Mom—and I called to tell her so. Over the phone line, I could hear it in her voice: She was thrilled. Without recriminations or regrets, she welcomed my overture. And I cried for relief, grateful that it wasn't too late for me to try to rebuild our bond.

Although Mom and Dad lived far away, Paul and I visited them as often as we could, sharing the highs and lows of parenting and grandparenting as our daughters Cara and Aster grew up. For me, forging a new connection with Mom and being able to share my life with her felt like a real-life miracle. I felt, and I still feel, that it was crucial to my success as a person.

Now I sit by Mom's bed, watching her quiet, careful breaths.

When her nurse Charlotte comes with medications or water, she lifts Mom up, squirts the liquid into her mouth and says, "Helen, can you try to swallow?" Amazingly, a few seconds later Mom's deeply carved Adam's apple slowly bobs up, then down—like a mechanical demonstration of how the human throat works. Mom's expression doesn't change.

The only time she indicates any distress is when Charlotte puts a small spoonful of orange ice cream in her mouth.

"It'll melt, so she can swallow it," Charlotte murmurs. But then Mom's shoulders shudder.

"Is she choking?" I ask, alarmed.

Mom gives a low, protesting moan—the only sound she's made since I arrived. We watch tensely. Finally she relaxes; evidently the ice cream has gone down.

"Do you think I should try another bite?" Charlotte asks doubtfully.

I shake my head. It would be too horrible if Mom choked, and food is no use now anyway.

Her time is measured in days, maybe hours. She's on her own timetable. I can't change that.

I have to go home tomorrow morning. I don't know what to wish for. I want to be with Mom when she dies, but I don't want her to die before she's ready.

After all this time, we have no unfinished business—except this. So I do the only thing I can do: I sit with Mom, waiting and remembering.

About the author: Diane Guernsey is the executive editor of Pulse—voices from the heart of medicine. *The morning after this piece was written, Diane's mother quietly passed away, with Diane at her bedside.*

An Intern's Guilt

Anna Kaltsas
12/12/2009

"She's been here for two months already. She's very complicated; you're going to be spending a lot of time with her and her family," my fellow intern said as she began signing out her patients to me.

It was my first rotation in the medical intensive care unit, and I was terrified. I was in my first few months as a "real" practicing physician—a title that I still felt uncomfortable with. When a nurse called out "Doctor!" I wouldn't respond, thinking that she couldn't possibly be referring to me.

My fear mushroomed as my co-intern rattled off the patient's problem list—bone-marrow transplant, shock liver, congestive heart failure, anemia, coagulopathy, sepsis, acute renal failure, ICU neuropathy, encephalopathy, ventilator-dependent...I knew what these meant, I just felt overwhelmed to see them all in a single patient.

Her name was Laura. Her story was impossibly tragic. A newly married, successful young professional, she'd visited her general practitioner two months back, complaining of weight loss and a headache, only to have blood tests reveal devastating news: leukemia.

Her first inpatient chemotherapy treatments had been followed by a bone-marrow transplant, then by complications from chemotherapy. A barrage of serious infections had landed her in the ICU.

Swollen with fluids as a result of her heart and kidney failure, Laura was thirty pounds over her normal weight. Chemotherapy had taken her hair. As her liver function worsened, her skin turned golden yellow, then bronze. Soon she developed oozing sores caused by edema and malnutrition (because her body couldn't absorb needed nutrients). The sores became infected, turning black-green. As her blood stopped clotting effectively, her skin became mottled with blood oozing from subcutaneous capillaries.

She had tubes everywhere—to feed her and help her breathe, to monitor her blood pressure and heart function, to help her urinate—even a rectal tube to help with her near-constant diarrhea.

Perhaps mercifully, Laura had been rendered unconscious by the multiple processes that caused toxins to build up in her blood and that reduced blood flow to her brain. The neurologists called it "toxic metabolic encephalopathy."

At first she was no more than a body and a collection of numbers to me; the machines told me what I needed to know to keep her alive. Yet, somehow, despite Laura's enfeebled, comatose state, a sense of her personality and life crept into my awareness.

One day, with a shock, I noticed on the windowsill a picture of her, smiling—probably placed there many weeks earlier by her mother. Laura was beautiful, with shiny blonde hair, gleaming white teeth, perfect porcelain skin. I walked in one morning to find her mother filing and painting her toenails, and then one evening I found her painfully attractive husband reading to her from a David Sedaris book. I cried on the phone to my mother that night, realizing that if I were ever in Laura's crushing situation, she would surely come tend to me in the same way.

I heard from the nurses that, prior to chemotherapy, Laura's biggest concern had been that she be able to freeze her eggs so that she could one day conceive a child. But once she was diagnosed, there was no time. She'd come to our hospital right away so that the leukemia could be treated.

Life with Laura was a roller-coaster. If her white count went up a tenth of a point, I ran to tell her husband and her mother. If her platelet count didn't respond to the latest transfusion, I somberly told them of the need for another one. Dutifully, I informed them when antibiotics were changed, when new consults were called and when the blood cultures indicated yet another life-threatening infection to be dealt with.

When my last night call arrived, I felt happy—happy to be leaving the next day, happy that I'd survived, and relieved that Laura would not die on my watch. The hematologists had told me to give her a platelet transfusion if her count fell under 10,000—the level below which the chances of a life-threatening bleed into the brain would increase substantially. On her evening labs, her count was 13,000. Per the instructions, I didn't transfuse her and ordered routine morning labs.

The nurse interrupted me at 5:00 in the morning as I was writing an admission note. "I think you'd better come and examine Laura. One pupil is dilated, and she's not breathing above the ventilator."

I walked to her room, my legs weak, and began to assess Laura's condition. My heart sank with each finding: one pupil "blown," wide-open and unreactive; no gag reflex; no spontaneous breaths. I called the supervising resident, then numbly listened to her directions: Order a head CT, then transfuse blood products to prevent further bleeding....

But I couldn't order the CT scan. When I sat down at the computer, my hands were shaking too much. The resident had to type the order for me.

Yet the reality of what had happened didn't sink in until the attending physician came onto the unit for morning rounds and said, "I'm so sorry, your patient is brain-dead."

I had to leave the room and get away from the shocked eyes of the ICU nurses, my colleagues and the attending—mortified that I couldn't keep the tears from streaming down my face.

The attending tried to console me, assuring me that this was the best that could have happened to Laura, that it was something he had prayed for. He also said that, had I not been caring for her, she wouldn't have lived as long as she did.

It didn't help.

I went home, relieved not to have to give Laura's family explanations or face their grief, glad to have the chance to be alone, yet churning with guilt over not having transfused her.

It's six years later, and I'm now the age Laura was when she received her diagnosis. I've had the chance to make and learn from my mistakes as a young physician; I've spent enough time in the ICU and in oncology units to become accustomed to death's inevitability, even at times to view it dispassionately. And yet, although an autopsy showed that my decision not to transfuse Laura wasn't the sole reason for her intracranial hemorrhage, I still can't shake the strong emotions that surface when I think of her.

I wonder if these emotions are brought on by lingering guilt over not having transfused her. Or do they reflect how much, in her youth and aspirations, Laura reminded me of myself—of my own good fortune, my own mortality?

About the author: Anna Kaltsas is currently pursuing a fellowship in infectious diseases at Montefiore Medical Center in the Bronx. She has maintained her interest in writing ever since her days as an undergraduate English literature major and has pursued it further through her ethics courses in medical school.

Babies

Elizabeth Szewczyk
12/18/2009

She tells me she wants to have a baby,
my daughter who was my baby
so many years ago.

Everything comes back to me—
the waiting, the wanting, the whisking
off to baby-earth, that angelic place,
passing through life
with its normal sounds, smells, and sights,
into the realm of women's starlight, bright
as Polaris, a celestial universe of power,
revolving so far away
that only women with growing
babies under their swollen, milk-gorged breasts
could inhabit this land.

Just for a moment, I want to have a baby again.
My aging body with its downhill breasts
and lost uterus aches to soar to that planet.
I want to feel life inside wiggle its
bowed, floppy legs, delicate arms,
those rubbery appendages not yet knit together.
I want to feel it somersault at
the top ledge of my ribs, understand
that surprising quiet of knowing
something inside me will come...
without him.

Just for a moment I want
every muscle in my baby-battered
body to unite for the same cause,
fold itself into my core, let
the sweet rush of sweat ambush my body,

the head opening me, dilating veins, stretching me
until I'm hollow,
our smells and bloods mixing together.
Just for a moment. Only one moment.

About the poet: Elizabeth Szewczyk, a recipient of the Connecticut Celebration of Excellence Award for writing, is the author of My Bags Were Always Packed: A Mother's Journey Through Her Son's Cancer Treatment and Remission. *Her poem "Birth" won first place in the literary journal* Shapes, *and her work has appeared in a number of poetry journals, including* Freshwater *and* Sanskrit. *Her first book of poetry,* This Becoming, *was published by Big Table Publishing. She teaches English at Asnuntuck Community College in Enfield, CT.*

About the poem: "'Babies' was written two years ago for my oldest daughter. She expressed the desire to start a family, and the poem grew from that one thought."

winter

pulse readers' hopes and wishes for the new year

Pulse *Readers*
1/1/2010

Editor's Note: We invited Pulse *readers to share with us their hopes and wishes for the New Year. Here are some of their responses.*

For my young patients who are living with HIV, I hope for relief from the stigma that shadows their lives, their health and their futures, and for acceptance and respect from family, friends, schools and society. For youth growing up surrounded by violence and poverty and by systems of education, health and human services that often fail them, I wish for empowering systems, safe spaces and nurturing adults who will help them to dream and to realize their potential.

Cathy Samples
(Director, Boston HAPPENS Program at Children's Hospital Boston)
Boston, MA

After watching my daughters experience three miscarriages, my wish (and prayer) for the new year is a healthy grandchild. My oldest daughter is now six weeks pregnant, and her first ultrasound is next week. We're praying this little one arrives in August, healthy and whole. What greater gift and wish is there than new life?

Elizabeth Szewczyk
Enfield, CT

I wish that today's medical students would become the healthcare reformers of tomorrow, taking the lead in controlling medical costs by practicing medicine that is science- and evidence-based and that includes best practices of prevention and health promotion. I wish that more medical school graduates would help to improve the health of the poor in their communities, in our nation and in nations beyond our borders. I wish that the students in my medical school would become tomorrow's physician advocates for social justice. I hope to maintain the energy and commitment needed to help today's medical students realize these possibilities.

Albert S. Kuperman
(Senior Advisor, Office of the Dean
Albert Einstein College of Medicine)
Bronx, NY

Haiku

Napa sparkling wine
truffled popcorn with butter—
first walk of the year

Neal Whitman
Pacific Grove, CA

I wish for healthy happiness in my life, for my family and friends, for my patients, for our community and for all the world. Peace and joy built on a foundation of health for all!

Kohar Jones
Chicago, IL

Nkosi Sikeleli Africa (God Bless Africa). These Xhosa words, an old hymn adopted as the national anthem of South Africa, are now more meaningful than ever. Bring an end to hatred, violence, intolerance, war, genocide, starvation and the scourge of AIDS and all else that may ravage this beautiful continent and its remarkable people. May the world see the beauty in this land and in the hearts and souls of her people and be emboldened by an overwhelming desire to save her. We are a part of Africa, and Africa is a part of us.

Patricia Lenahan
(Director, Comprehensive CARE Center
Share Our Selves—SOS)
Costa Mesa, CA

Peace on earth
Good will toward men
Affordable health care for all

Jeri Burn
South Lyon, MI

I dream and hope for change beyond healthcare reform. Let there be healing with touch, talk and, yes, of course, medicine.

Katherine Ellington
Saint Albans, NY

- I wish our EMR (electronic medical record) weren't so awful!!!

- And that someone would discover a cure for traffic...and inconsiderateness...crowds...and stupidity.

- (I wish that I could learn to frame my realities less negatively.)

- I wish that I were smarter, fitter, faster, wittier...or that others were less discriminating about these matters...or believed that the way I am represents the ideal.

- I wish that when I wished for the end of ALL world suffering, it didn't sound like such a cliché...or seem like overcompensating for being self-absorbed.

- I wish that I had ignored the invitation to wish in the first place...or at least had done a better job with the opportunity.

Sean C. Lucan
Bronx, NY

Haiku

That all whose cup runs
over see it, fill those whose
cups are underfilled.

Robert S. Fawcett
(Associate Director
York Hospital Family Medicine Residency)
York, PA

May this year bring each of us the blessing of honoring our feelings and experiences, accepting ourselves in all our complexity, integrating our wounds with our gifts and deeply enjoying the moments of our lives.

Ronit Fallek
New York, NY

I wish that key stakeholders, numerous and diverse as they are, would work collaboratively towards resolving the formidable health-related issues that we face in this nation. I wish that the health care provided to individuals would encompass sensitivity and compassion and extend to families, care-givers and their communities. I wish that healthcare practitioners would renew their commitment and find a genuine sense of meaning and fulfill-ment in their critically important work.

Diane M. Kondratowicz
(Coordinator, Patient-centered Medicine Scholars Program
University of Illinois College of Medicine at Chicago)
Chicago, IL

I wish that more and more people will reach out to those in need and realize that giving is what brings us happiness.

Xinshu She
(Albert Einstein College of Medicine
Johns Hopkins School of Public Health)
Baltimore, MD

A Haiku Dream for 2010

Golden, smiling suns
Days of wonder, good health, love
Star-filled nights of peace

Ronna Edelstein
Pittsburgh, PA

It is most certainly a time in history for an era of compassion, integrity and safety. Let's begin with medicine and blaze the trail in 2010. The others will follow when they see our success.

Dale Ann Micalizzi
(Executive Director, Justin's HOPE Project
The Task Force for Global Health)
Schenectady, NY

I wish that everyone who wants to conceive will be successful at bringing new life into this world and that no one will need to know the pain of infertility.

Paula M. Zimlicki
Menlo Park, CA

Here's wishing everyone affordable health coverage, a warm house to live in and good, healthy food to eat.

Brenda Caronia
Bronx, NY

For my first-year medical students, I wish that their interest in patients as persons continues into next year. For my second-year students, I hope that when they enter their clerkships in the summer they will remember what they learned about humanism and will still think of Mrs. Mary Jones as a patient in room 210 and not as "the gallbladder in 210."

Maurice Bernstein
(Keck School of Medicine
University of Southern California)
Los Angeles, CA

Reflections from a senior citizen

Dorothy Kligerman
1/8/2010

I used to talk of fun and games
Now I talk of aches and pains.
I used to paint the town bright red
Now at nine I am in bed.

I used to dream of lovers bold.
Now if truth be told
The only men who interest me
Are those with a medical degree.

"Why," you ask, "have they such clout?"
Well—we have so much to talk about:
There's my arthritis and stenosis,
Hypertension, scoliosis.

In a cozy room, alone, we chat.
We never have a lover's spat.
So keep your handsome Romeos
I'll always take those medicos!

———————————

About the poet: *Dorothy Kligerman died on August 30, 2011, at the age of ninety-six. She is greatly missed by family and friends for her loving heart, quick wit and indomitable spirit. At the time her poem was published online in* Pulse, *Dorothy provided the following biography: "I am ninety-five years old, widowed, with three married children, four grandchildren and two great-grandchildren. My first published work appeared in February, 1931, in* The Record Book *of my graduating class of Simon Gratz High School in Philadelphia. It was not until the 1980s that my work appeared in print again. I was a reporter for the* Mt. Airy Express, *writing on assignment twice monthly and actually being paid! The paper folded at the end of that decade. Again there was a hiatus, until in 2006 I enrolled at TARP (Temple Association for Retired Persons), sponsored by Temple University, which offered many classes for senior citizens. I chose the Poetry Workshop, led by the energetic and inspirational Peggy Walsh McKenna. I am grateful to her."*

About the poem: *"At ninety-five, I do have aches and pains, and I am grateful to all of my doctors for keeping me well."*

May I Have Your Attention, Please?

Adam Philip Stern
1/15/2010

Some sentences should never be interrupted.

"We have the results of your HIV test," the attending physician had begun. But fate interrupted with a seemingly endless loudspeaker announcement:

"May I have your attention, please? Would the following patients please report to the nurse's station for morning medications...."

Nothing about Benjamin's story was ordinary. He had been voluntarily admitted to an inpatient psychiatry unit after reporting many symptoms of depression—extreme somnolence, fatigue, thirty-pound weight loss with poor appetite, diffuse pain, decreased energy and joylessness for about three months.

Benjamin was charming, smart and eager to follow medical advice. As a relatively inexperienced medical student, I found interviewing him a refreshing change of pace from my difficult interactions with the poorly groomed individuals who paced the halls repeating nonsensical phrases and questions over and over again. Benjamin always peppered our talks with comments about current events and informed questions about his care. He could often be seen reading the newspaper or interacting with other patients or staff in a way that made me wonder whether he really belonged there.

Benjamin's life story was as engaging as his demeanor. He had worked as a city fire fighter for about thirty years before injuring his leg on the job—an injury that brought him chronic pain and an early retirement.

More dramatically, after twenty years of marriage Benjamin had come out as a gay man. He'd then proceeded to engage in unprotected sex with multiple partners.

With so many physical complaints, including weight loss and low energy, we had to wonder whether some of his symptoms, including the depression itself, might be manifestations of HIV infection. But I was reassured when he told me that he had tested negative just two months prior. We performed the test anyway, knowing that it would be days before we'd get the results, and continued treating him as a simple case of depression.

Over the next week, Benjamin responded well to antidepressants, and one day the entire treatment team agreed that he was ready for discharge the following morning. We informed him and prepared his paperwork. That evening I checked the computer for any new lab results. The screen read, "HIV antibody test: Positive, confirmed with Western Blot."

This must be a mistake, I thought. Then feelings of despair and disappointment crept over me.

The news felt like a punch in the stomach; it was also a logistical nightmare. My attending physician suggested that I inform the patient that we'd need to do some more tests before his discharge (to figure out how advanced his HIV was). We would tell him his diagnosis in the morning.

Excuse me? So, as the least experienced person on the team, I'm supposed to tell the patient that he won't be discharged as planned and that we need more blood tests, without giving him any hint about his new diagnosis or what the blood tests are for?

Noting my obvious distress, my supervising resident joined me on the long journey to the patient's room and took the lead in discussing the situation with him. Very casually, he mentioned that we would need to do a few more tests before he could be discharged. Benjamin nodded stoically.

"I understand," he said knowingly.

The next morning, with the team gathered, the patient walked down the corridor to the "music room" at a snail's pace. He looked like someone on his way to the electric chair. I wondered if on some level he knew about the news he was about to receive. Were his slow steps an attempt to hold onto his happy innocence as long as possible? As for me, I found myself walking faster than usual despite my best efforts to seem casual.

When everyone had finally gathered, the attending began his well-rehearsed talk. When he arrived at the punchline and the loudspeaker interrupted him, I couldn't bear to make eye contact with anyone—not the attending, holding up a finger to signal patience, and not Benjamin, who seemed to be handling the situation far more gracefully than I.

The announcement lasted for what felt like the longest fifteen seconds of my life, then the attending resumed:

"The test came back positive."

Benjamin closed his eyes and sat perfectly still. I waited for any kind of emotional reaction, but none came. What followed was a very ordinary conversation about what these results meant and how they would affect his life. Benjamin, staring at the floor, said that he wished he'd been more careful and added that perhaps he hadn't been tested in recent months as he'd thought. He thanked us and finally smiled in my direction as if to tell me that everything would be all right.

I felt myself exhale.

My experience with Benjamin taught me that, in medicine, roles can get blurred and near-certainties turned upside-down in moments. I now have a better sense of why doctors so often distance themselves emotionally from their patients' outcomes; the alternative is to feel the awful hurt that I felt when I came face-to-face with Benjamin's diagnosis.

Yet I'm glad that I got to know Benjamin, talked openly with him—and cared enough to ache. I will carry that experience with me for the rest of my career.

About the author: *Adam Philip Stern is a third-year resident with Harvard Longwood Psychiatry Residency Training Program in Boston, MA. When he wrote this story, he was a fourth-year medical student at SUNY Upstate Medical*

University. "I have written creatively for as long as I can remember and hope that writing will make me a better doctor even as medicine makes me a better writer." Adam's novella The Insatiable Man is available through online booksellers, and his fiction has been published in The Healing Muse, Lifelines, Harmony Magazine, Blood and Thunder and The Rejected Quarterly.

confessions of a seventy-five-year-old drug addict

Arlene Silverman
1/22/2009

The physician, a slim young man with a shaved head and intense, dark eyes, reaches out to shake hands. I fumble to extend one hand while the other clutches a questionnaire that I haven't finished filling out.

"That's okay," Dr. Gordon says. "You can finish later."

He can tell that I'm nervous, but seems to understand. He knows that I've had to sign in at a window surrounded by other patients, many younger than my own children. Some of them look dazed; others have dozed off. Still others, alert, look as if they'd just come from their job at the bank.

Me? I walk with a cane. My clothes have been carefully chosen to look presentable. I've come through a door labeled "Chemical Dependency Clinic" in small, discreet letters. If you hadn't been looking for the sign, you'd have missed it. The building has no street-level windows and is in a neighborhood that could kindly be called "transitional," rundown at its core but reluctantly yielding to gentrification.

I am seventy-five years old, and I have come to Dr. Gordon because I've become addicted to drugs.

While he scrolls through my lengthy records on the computer, I flip through the questionnaire. Do I drink alcohol? (Barely.) Am I depressed? (Often.) Do I ever feel suicidal? (Well, I guess not—but maybe. Don't we all sometimes?)

Dr. Gordon brings out a breathalyzer to measure my alcohol level. "Sorry, it's a requirement," he says.

I tell him my story.

Five months ago, I fractured my pelvis in two places, the result of a fall suffered when the theater "popcorn guy" showed me to my seat after the movie had started—and there was no seat there.

"From that moment on, I felt pain as I'd never known it," I say. "After x-rays at the hospital, I was transferred to a nursing home and was immediately put on pain medication."

"What kind?" asks Dr. Gordon.

"A fentanyl patch," I say. "I was complaining about extreme pain." The patch was started at fifty micrograms, I recall, but was increased over time until, by the time I left, I'd "graduated" to 125. "They sent me home with a prescription for Percocet and those patches."

"When did you notice a problem?" Dr. Gordon asks.

"When I got home. The pelvic fractures were healing, so I wanted to feel like myself again and not depend on drugs. Despite my daughter's warnings—she's a nurse—I started to downgrade the dose of the patch, figuring it would make my recovery go faster." What no one had explained to me is that fentanyl, an opiate, is fifty to 100 times more potent than morphine and can be addictive.

I found out just how addictive the hard way. Not having been told how to lower the dose, I went at it too quickly and ended up in an emergency room with withdrawal symptoms.

"I sat for three hours waiting to be seen," I say. "I couldn't stay still. I kept putting my head in my daughter's lap. It was how I imagine the worst flu to be. Finally they gave me morphine and sent me home."

Dr. Gordon glances at the record and says, "You were prescribed Percocet to withdraw from the fentanyl." Percocet—oxycodone—is another opiate.

"I'm here," I say, "because now I'm addicted to Percocet."

I tell him about bothering my physician for more frequent prescriptions and about waiting anxiously, like a wino craving a drink, for my son to return from the pharmacy with my next supply of pills.

"I'm trying to withdraw on my own, but my nights are, well, nightmares. I shake, my legs flail all over the bed, I can't sleep," I say. My primary-care physician told me to "bite the bullet," that I will get better. A psychiatrist sent me to group therapy for addicts and gave me various tranquilizers, including Ativan, Risperdol and Seroquel. But the misery lingers.

With a feeble attempt at humor, I say, "If I'm going to be a drug addict, at least I should enjoy it."

I tell Dr. Gordon that I'm reminded of that nursery rhyme about the old lady who swallowed a fly, then a spider to catch the fly. ("Perhaps she'll die.")

Dr. Gordon seems both sympathetic and worried. "Addiction isn't only a problem for young people," he says. "It's growing among seniors."

There's sort of a war going on in the field of pain management, he continues. One camp worries about opiate addiction; the other is more concerned about the effects of long-term pain. It seems that, given my pain's severity, my doctors opted for opiates.

Dr. Gordon then hands me a day-by-day timetable of gradual Percocet withdrawal and clonidine tablets to counteract the withdrawal symptoms, assuring me that clonidine is not addictive. The last thing I want, I tell him, is to get addicted to yet another drug. ("There was an old lady who swallowed a bird....")

Eventually, my pelvis heals, although even now my gait sometimes resembles that of a very old Frankenstein.

And I finally kick the Percocet habit.

In some ways, though, I will never be the same. I'm more wary, less resilient. Even though I've always considered myself independent, I know now that the slightest waver in the orbit of my life can send it off course.

I still ask myself: Why wasn't I strong enough to handle the pain? Handle the drugs? Did I do something wrong? Did I not bite the bullet hard enough?

Most of all, I regret having missed the chance to avoid all of this. What should I have asked the doctors at the nursing home? What should they have told me about the heavy-duty drugs I was taking?

And what about the doctor-patient communications that never happened, but that might have made things turn out differently? The doctor prescribes. The patient follows instructions. It's a neat paper transaction. No questions asked on either side.

Finally, there's something else that bothers me.

One substance-abuse expert has called addiction among elders "the silent epidemic." How long, I wonder, before that waiting room at the Chemical Dependency Clinic is filled with people like me?

———————————

About the author: Arlene Silverman, a San Francisco-based writer, started contributing to local publications when her children were small. Since then, her articles have appeared in the San Francisco Chronicle, Christian Science Monitor, Saturday Evening Post, Newsweek ("My Turn") *and other publications. In the past, she has worked as a teacher, parent-involvement coordinator and grant writer. At present, she is very happy while in the company of her four grandchildren.*

médecins sans frontières — Liberia, 2003

Les Cohen
1/29/2010

I walk warily,
searching for life
through smoking remains
of a jungle village.

My flashlight beam
slices the black haze
of equatorial darkness.
Was it Suakoko?
Fokwelleh?

No wind, rustle or drum
pierces the silence
of West African night.
Torched husks of thatched huts,
clay walls liquefied,
charred dog skeletons,
feet outstretched
as if running from Hell.
Stench of burnt flesh pervades,
stinging eyes and nostrils.

Soft footsteps coming close.
A small, thin boy approaches;
mahogany face, bright teeth
glisten in the moonlight.
Bloody machete, strings of
bleached-white finger
bones dangle over a tattered

ARMY OF ETERNAL PEACE
T-shirt.

Smiling, voice soft,
he hisses
Give me medsuh,
give me cokayh,
mistah.

No, no,
don't kill me,
I am doctuh,
take my medical bag, wallet, watch, shoes.
I try to scream, but
no sound escapes.

He slowly lifts an AK-47
to my face.
Shaking his head, grinning
his finger curls,
tightening around the trigger.

About the poet: Les Cohen has taught and practiced in Boston for many years. His short stories have appeared in The Cleveland Clinic Journal of Medicine, The Yale Journal of Humanities in Medicine, Annals of Internal Medicine, Archives of Internal Medicine, Journal of General Internal Medicine, JAMA, Hospital Drive *and* r.kv.r.y *quarterly literary journal.*

About the poem: "I was a Peace Corps physician in Liberia from 1965 to 1967. In 2003, when I saw a photograph of one of the smiling 'soldiers' of Taylor's Children's Army and read of the courageous work of MSF, I wrote this prose poem."

postmortem

Sandy Brown
2/5/2010

Coming out of my exam room on a Monday morning, I saw two overweight police officers standing in my waiting room. From past experience, I knew that they were there to tell me that one of my patients had died and to collect information for the coroner's report. Even as I geared up to hear the impending bad news, the doctor in me couldn't help wondering how they'd passed their department physicals.

"Do I need to call a lawyer?" I joked, trying to guess which of my patients it could be.

"Michael Freund died on Saturday," said Dalia, my office manager.

It was a shot to my gut. Mike was seventy-three years old, but one of my healthiest patients for his age. He neither smoked nor drank, took no medicines except for the occasional Viagra and played tennis with a passion. He was fit and trim, and I couldn't imagine what had done him in.

I hadn't seen Mike in the months since he'd come in for his annual exam, which had raised no red flags. Then I remembered that he had called me the previous Thursday with some vague complaint that I couldn't recall. I'd set him up for an appointment the next day, but he'd called to cancel, telling Dalia he was feeling better.

Now, three days later, he was dead.

The police weren't much help, except to say that he'd had collapsed while doing something or other, and that an autopsy was pending. They copied what they needed from his chart and walked out, leaving me to ponder the cause of death—and awash in emotions.

In addition to being my patient, Mike was my friend. He had come to me six years earlier as a Bay Area refugee looking for a life in the country. Learning that he was both a handyman and an artist, I had him do some repair work around my office. My building has joists cantilevering out to support a deck, and they'd been attacked by rot from the deck. I'd thought that the whole deck would have to be torn down and rebuilt, but Mike had Sawzalled away the bad wood, like a surgeon debriding a wound, and scabbed on good wood using lots of glue and paint. Another time, when a putrid odor permeated the office, he'd squeezed through a crawl space to see if there was a dead critter under the floor. Not finding any, he'd concluded that something had died in the walls; we simply had to wait for it to dessicate until the smell finally went away. Not many patients would get down and dirty for you like Mike did.

I couldn't wait to get the autopsy report—what had I missed?—so I called the county coroner for a preliminary read. The secretary was helpful; the cause of death, she said, was "cardiac ischemia," meaning an insufficient blood supply to the heart.

That struck me as odd, but odder still was to get the report a few days later and find no internal exam results. It was as though the pathologist's "autopsy" had consisted of simply glancing at Mike's body. Nothing had been checked beneath the skin—no body cavity explored, no organs weighed or examined. Surely they'd accidentally omitted the internal exam from the transcript; could the pathologist actually have neglected to do it? This procedure wouldn't even pass for an autopsy on television, where they get all the medical stuff wrong. My calls to the coroner went unreturned, and I was left wondering if this was their standard operating procedure or just an aberration.

Mike's newspaper obituary mentioned that a celebration of his life was to be held at his home the next Saturday. I don't go to many of these affairs; if someone dies, I worry that people will hold the doctor responsible. Maybe I *was* responsible—maybe I should have paid more attention to a patient who was likely minimizing his symptoms in an effort to fool himself.

Try as I might, I couldn't remember why Mike had wanted to see me. His call had come as I was leaving for the day; I'd scheduled him without even noting his complaint, probably because it didn't sound serious. And when he didn't show, I hadn't thought much of it. Was that negligent of me? I would have given anything to have recorded that last conversation. Anyhow, I decided to go to Mike's celebration.

Arriving at his house, I met Vicki, his girlfriend of two years, who lived in a nearby town.

"Mike told me he'd canceled his appointment with you," she said. "He was having bad reflux, but then he felt better. He came over on Saturday, then he went to play tennis while I went shopping. He played three hard sets with younger players and beat them all. After the match, he collapsed. They say he had a heart attack. His father died of one when he was forty-six, but his brother is still alive at eighty-two, so Mike figured he hadn't gotten the bad genes."

I didn't remember Mike's family history quite that way. As I recalled, his father had died of congestive heart failure at sixty-two. But I wasn't going to argue the point. Besides, he'd had no other cardiac risks or complaints.

I walked around Mike's house, looking at all his artwork. He was prolific; there were abstract paintings everywhere. Several tennis rackets lay on the floor of his bedroom. Once, he'd given me one to get me to play with him. Sadly, that had never happened....

As his tennis-playing and art-world friends began to arrive, I left.

I didn't want to be introduced as Mike's doctor.

About the author: Sandy Brown practices family and preventive medicine in Fort Bragg, CA. For more than six years he wrote the column "Practice Diary" for Family Practice Management, parts of which were translated in the Chinese Journal of General Practice. He now writes for Medscape Family Medicine as well as facilitating their family-medicine and internal-medicine discussion boards. When not writing or seeing patients, he enjoys dirt and mountain bike riding, counseling premeds about how to get into medical school and advocating for independent practice.

keeping secrets

Reeta Mani
2/12/2010

Rohit walked into our HIV-testing center in South Mumbai one busy morning. I was struck by how stylish he looked in his jeans and casual linen shirt, very different than the usual patients who visit our sprawling public hospital campus. He paced back and forth in a corner, looking at his watch and whispering into a cell phone.

I guessed that he'd chosen this crowded setting because of the anonymity it afforded; here he stood little risk of running into an acquaintance who might start to wonder.

During Rohit's pre-test counseling, he confided his fear of being HIV-positive. He told us about having unprotected sex with female commercial sex workers during overseas business trips—and about a routine insurance health checkup that had hinted at something wrong.

He was here to learn the truth.

The next day, when he came for his results, Rohit was astonishingly calm.

"Your blood sample has tested positive for HIV," I said and, per our routine, handed him the lab report so he could see for himself.

Rohit held the piece of paper and sat, gazing deeply into nowhere. Just when I thought he might have a million questions, he forced a smile and abruptly stood up. "Thank you, Ma'am," he said, avoiding my gaze, and was gone in an instant.

A week later he came back, as we'd asked, bringing his wife Anjali.

I was prepared to meet a meek, submissive housewife. Instead, Anjali was an attractive executive who worked for a well-known multinational corporation. She came across as independent and confident, yet she also had a childlike naïveté that made me want to reach out to her. As our counselor Neha and I sat with her, Anjali told us how devastated she'd been by Rohit's diagnosis.

And there was more.

Except for the first few years of their marriage, Rohit and she had never really gotten along. Rohit had always been suspicious of her business trips with male colleagues. She'd tried to convince him of her innocence, but to no avail. The real issue, she suspected, was that Rohit's male ego was threatened by her successful career.

It took a lot of coaxing before Anjali would herself agree to be tested for HIV.

"I was furious at Rohit when he broke the news to me," she said. "I felt betrayed, hurt, angry with myself, lonely, depressed—all at once. I even wanted to end my life." Her eyes welled with tears. "Can you please tell me this isn't true? That it's just a bad dream?" She began sobbing uncontrollably.

"Anjali," I said gently, "we have no doubt about Rohit's test results. The sooner you can accept it, the easier it will be for all of us to deal with."

"Yes," she answered. "I have to live to care for Rohit, to cherish the memory of the wonderful times we spent together, to forgive him for a mistake he committed, probably in a stray moment when he wasn't himself...."

As Anjali spoke I glanced over at Rohit, seated outside, without a hint of regret in his eyes. I felt fury rising inside me.

Here was a woman with beauty, brains and a high-profile job. This man had virtually destroyed her life, yet she wanted to forgive him and devote herself to him! She was acting as if she were God. Or, muttered an inner voice, just plain stupid.

Anjali's test came back positive for HIV.

In some ways, she was like so many of the women we see here, day in and day out, women infected by their husbands, whom they had trusted unquestioningly.

When we broke the news to Anjali and Rohit, we expected a verbal blame-game. But they surprised us again: Each seemed to want to act as the other's emotional anchor.

We told them that, although no cure for HIV currently exists, with regular treatment and follow-up, appropriate nutrition, exercise and a positive attitude, they could lead healthy lives. Both discussed the treatment options. As Rohit gently held Anjali's hand and helped her out of her seat, they seemed geared up to fight the disease together.

I couldn't help but note that, although the ecstasy of independence had torn them apart, the agony of suffering had drawn them closer. Ironically, HIV had given their marriage a new lease on life.

As Rohit and Anjali left to start therapy at another hospital, I felt oddly happy for them. HIV had snatched away the arrogance born of freedom and was instead fostering mutual reliance. I hoped that they would continue to seek, nurture and cherish their love for one another—a love that had seemed lost beyond recall.

I found myself smiling as an unlikely thought came to mind: Every cloud has a silver lining!

Postscript:

The story did not quite end here.

There are two types of HIV virus: HIV-1 and HIV-2. While doing further testing for research purposes, we found that Rohit had been infected with the HIV-2 virus, and Anjali with HIV-1. Apparently they had each acquired the infection from a different source! It looked as if someone other than Rohit had infected Anjali.

Were his suspicions of her well-founded after all?

I never found out. In fact, I never saw Rohit and Anjali again. We considered calling them to inform them about this new twist in the plot, but after much deliberation decided against it. I wasn't sure that this new information would be helpful to them. How many more skeletons were waiting to tumble out of the closet?

More than that, I didn't want to shatter their fragile relationship, now held together by shared sorrow. Their decision to battle HIV together seemed to have united them.

And so I chose, in the end, to let it be.

About the author: Reeta Mani is a virologist at the National Institute of Mental Health and Neurosciences (NIMHANS) in Bangalore, India. "Since childhood I have always loved to write. My profession earns me my bread and butter, but as a writer I have the freedom to express what I cannot possibly as a doctor, fettered by decorum, scientific reasoning, political correctness and ethics."

death at a distance

Edwin Gardiner
2/19/2010

Your message hung on the phone line
like his striped shirt blowing
in the last wind of his life:
softly and with dignity.
His facial bones,
and body contours
he allowed to be chiseled
to an insubstantial sharpness
by the flow of chemicals and
the relentless labor of his disease:
both polished his body to dust.
Your life that has breathed that dust
for years will, someday,
carry it to the stars,
where it belongs.

———————————

About the poet: *Edwin Gardiner, a urologist, was in private practice for thirty years in San Diego; he did his surgical training at UCSF and NYU-Bellevue Medical Center. "I've written since my undergraduate days at Amherst College but have had only essays and professional monographs published before. From the early 1980s on, I occasionally wrote poetry, but since retiring I've found poetics an essential part of sampling the temperature of my daily life. My recent poetry has focused on dealing with loss and the ironic emergence of humor in otherwise dark or dismal surroundings. It's like hearing a voice from under the stone whisper: 'What, you again? You look thin; try cooking instead of weeping!'"*

About the poem: *"The man in this poem and I were friends for many years. This poem was a whisper of condolence to his wife upon receiving a phone call with the news of his death. Though the poem is 'occasional' in the sense of being inspired by an event, the act of constructing it became a way for me to transform the sadness I felt, using the biological effects of dying to examine a more generalized transformation of biological matter into the balanced structure of the universe. With his wife as his lover and caretaker, I'm hinting at her related role as a messenger of this larger transformation of us all."*

The case of the screaming man

Paula Lyons
2/26/2010

As everyone knows, the human body has orifices. Occasionally, these become occluded, or occupied, by things that aren't supposed to be there. Every doctor knows this, as does almost everyone else. Who hasn't heard, as a child, the cautionary phrase "Don't stick beans up your nose"?

Human nature being what it is, almost every clinician must deal with foreign objects—flora, fauna—that have been put into places where they don't belong. Sometimes, though, "beans" can materialize without a patient's permission.

Here is one such case—a personal favorite of mine—that I've mentally entitled "The Screaming Man."

I was back in the furthermost part of the clinic, arguing with an insurance company representative about the need for a patient's CT scan, when one of our receptionists ran up.

"Dr. Lyons! There's a man screaming in the waiting room!"

"Is he bleeding?"

"No, he's banging his head with his hands and screaming! I think he might be crazy!"

I ran to the front. There in our packed waiting room was in fact a seemingly crazy man, screaming, dancing around and batting at his left ear with both hands. The other patients were cringing away from him, their eyes wide. He was burly, dressed in a City laborer's jumpsuit soiled with leaves and debris. With every leap, his heavy work boots left red mud clods on the floor.

"Jesus Christ, help me! Get it out! Get it OUT! It's MOVING!"

Okay, now I had a clue. I grabbed the man by his suit front, assured him that we would help and pulled him into an exam room, calling for the ear-nose-and-throat tray and some mineral oil.

When I looked through the otoscope into his left ear, I nearly screamed myself: Staring back at me were the multiple, horrifyingly enlarged eyes of a common spider. Probably equally terrified, it was clinging with all eight legs to the inside of this man's ear canal.

Now the cause of my patient's frenzy was clear. Once an arthropod (as the medical literature likes to call spiders and insects) makes its way into the human ear, every one of its tiny movements sounds as loud as a jet airplane to its unfortunate host. Add to this the creepy knowledge that your ear has been "invaded" by a creature that would make you recoil if you encountered it in the bathroom sink, and you have the perfect recipe for temporary insanity.

My patient, calming down a bit, explained that he had been clearing brush with one of his coworkers close behind and had felt a tickling sensation on top of his left ear. Suspecting a joke perpetrated by his coworker, he had swiped at the ear, only to feel the sensation of many wriggling feet running for cover, right into the nearest dark hole.

Now that I'd had a chance to assess the situation, I realized that only one of my two patients could survive. I chose to save the larger. A syringe of mineral oil, gently instilled, quickly euthanized the spider, and I washed the tiny carcass out of the man's ear with saline.

One part of me rejoiced at the relief in my human patient's face, now that he'd been freed from the tormenting interior flamenco dance. Another part of me wondered wryly if we should be playing "Taps" for the intrepid arachnid explorer.

The man insisted that I spread its draggled corpse with forceps so that he could make sure that none of the legs remained within his ear. Together, we counted all eight. Then he paused and reflected.

"Doc, you don't think it had time to lay eggs in there, do you?"

I hid my smile. "No, certainly not."

My patient began to recover his composure—and his swagger. He asked me to place the tiny body in a sterile urine container so he could show his friends the proof of his ordeal. By the time he left our clinic, amid the smiles and congratulations of the staff, I felt certain that, had the spider been just a bit larger, he would have had it stuffed and mounted.

The clinic staff and I went on to enjoy a long and congenial relationship with this patient—whose nickname forever after, of course, was "Spider Man."

About the author: Paula Lyons is a native of New Jersey who graduated from Emory University School of Medicine. She now practices family medicine just outside of Baltimore, MD. Some of her other writings have appeared in Pulse, The Pharos *and* The Journal of Family Practice.

family business

Joanne Wilkinson
3/5/2010

My mother's mother was more a force of nature than a person. Chablis in hand, stockings bagging a little over her solid, practical navy pumps, she delivered her opinions without the slightest sugar-coating. She used words like "simply" and "absolutely" a lot. "He is quite simply the worst mayor we've ever had." "She had absolutely no business having four children." My cousins and I all listened and quaked, hoping the wrath would not be turned on us. Even after my mother's death, when you might imagine she would soften toward me a little, I still felt the need to stand up straighter whenever she looked at me. Behind her back, I called her "The Graminator."

The Graminator had been retired for almost as long as I could remember and she had three major interests: wine, the stock ticker on CNN and the politics of the Catholic Church, upon which she delivered opinions at every party.

I thought of her almost like Scrooge, hoarding and counting her certainties while all the people she had alienated went out to eat together in a messy, shabby, second-rate fellowship of true happiness. I felt caught in the middle: I cared little about the stock ticker and felt her opinions were harsh, but I couldn't quite abandon myself to not caring what she thought of me.

For much of my adult life I have been haunted by a story she told me in my early childhood about heaven. Everyone would be questioned, she told me, as to what gifts they had been given, and how they had used them. "You have a lot of gifts," she told me sternly, looking over her glasses at my five-year-old self. "So it's even more important that you find a way to use each and every one. Wisely. *To help other people.*"

Many times, as I slogged through medical school and residency and wondered where the fun part was, I remembered this conversation, and thought wistfully about my friends who were contentedly taking over the family business—running a restaurant or doing carpentry or plumbing. Did they wake up at night wondering whether they were using all their special gifts the right way?

Although I barely remember her working, the Graminator was a career woman; she went back to grad school in the sixties, when her children were grown, and got her doctoral degree, writing her dissertation on the mainstreaming of mentally retarded children into the general classroom in elementary school. She then became a professor of psychology at a local college. I wonder, often, just how many students she terrorized the way she terrorized me.

Recently, having transitioned to a research career, I read her dissertation for the first time and was blown away by its concise and timely hypothesis and by the rigorous nature of the research. I sat with the yellowed pages in my hands and wondered, forty-five years too late, what journal she should have sent it to.

When my husband and I became engaged, we walked across the street to the Graminator's house so that she would be the first to know. (I thought she'd like that—the whole first-to-know business.) She sat perfectly still when we told her the news, then heaved a gusty sigh.

"Well, I wish you all the luck in the world," she said. "You know half of all marriages end in divorce these days." Chastened, we crunched back down the gravel driveway to my house.

"Should we call your mom next?" I asked my husband gingerly. By the time the wedding rolled around, dementia had seized the Graminator in its diminishing grip.

"You have a *husband*?" she would ask me incredulously after that, as though an alien spaceship had landed in my backyard and I had invited one of them in to live with me. "Are you *happy*?"

When my husband and I decided to adopt, I didn't make the same mistake twice. A few days before I flew to South America for our daughter, I visited the Graminator at her nursing home ("It's not a nursing home. It's an assisted-living facility," she would hiss) and told her I would be traveling a lot for work this fall, and not to worry if she didn't hear from me. I could only imagine what her pronouncements on adoption would be, particularly the adoption of a child whose skin might be darker than mine.

When I returned, however, many exhausting months later, Grammy was lit up with joy. "All these years," she told me, "I've been wondering why I am still alive—why hasn't God taken me yet? And now," she said, cradling my daughter's little head, "now I know why."

For months afterward, whenever we would visit the nursing home, Grammy would see us from the hallway as she participated in yoga, sing-along, bingo.

"Oh!" she would say, interrupting whoever she was talking to. "I have to go. That's my *great-granddaughter*."

One weekend this September, I got the call from my aunt that I had been expecting for years: the Graminator appeared to be in a coma, possibly from a stroke. Hospice was involved.

I visited her three times over four days, sat with her, talked to her, and read while she stared at the ceiling and her breath rattled in and out.

On the fourth day I returned to Boston, to work. There was nothing I could do for her, and she appeared not to know I was there, yet I was racked with guilt and indecision. I needed to work, I needed my daughter's schedule to be as normal as possible and for her to be safe and content, but I also wanted to be with my grandmother.

I realize on the second day of guilt that Grammy had been a working mother too. If anyone could understand how I felt that day, it would be her.

When the Graminator died two days later, the obituary that I wrote appeared in the local papers. It stressed her career accomplishments, her research and education in the field of elementary education for children with intellectual disabilities, and her mentorship of so many other teachers and advocates for the disabled.

It doesn't mention that, as it happens, my new research position involves funding from NIH to study cancer screening in adults with intellectual disabilities. I don't think Grammy realized this, nor did I when I started that job, but I wound up in the family business after all.

About the author: Joanne Wilkinson is an assistant professor of family medicine at the Boston University School of Medicine. Her short stories and essays have been published in the Journal of Family Practice, Family Medicine, Medicine & Health Rhode Island *and* Medical Economics. *She has won several awards for creative writing and in 2008 was awarded the Mid-Career Faculty Achievement Award by the Family Medicine Education Consortium. She lives in the Boston area with her family.*

in the pediatric ward

Tess Galati
3/12/2010

In this forest of tubes and bottles,
Children wander in sleep.
A dying bird drops
From the corner of my eye.
The night nurse floats through paths
Tending the rooted tubes,
Weighing the pause between breaths.
In the dark, a man's voice
Stuns like a hunter's gun.
We wait for dawn.

Last night we cried—four worn children
Facing their walls, and I,
Handing out animal crackers.
Willow's bones are flaking
John's eye refuses light
Paige's ears close up and
Something is eating the soft parts of
Adam's knee.
We know these things and we cry.

The children force the beds to do acrobatic tricks.
They've decorated the sheets with urine, gum, and ice cream.
Shrieking, they dribble gravy; Collages bloom on the floor.
They glue flies to the walls, punch holes in dolls and blankets.
The children are not civilized, and the women have left off makeup.

After the baths, the doctors
Visit their explanations
Upon the numbered beds.
They know about bones, eyes, ears,
For they've inspected the bodies.
They neither laugh nor cry.

We humor them, for we see
That their suits are too tight,
Their shoes pinch,
And they've had little sleep.

But at three in the morning,
Adam and Willow whimper,
Aquarium gurgles
IV fluid drips
Vibrators hum
A dying bird falls
And the night nurse's thighs
rub, rub in the hall.

About the poet: Tess Galati is a Greek immigrant who grew up in Iowa. At seventeen, she was sent back to the old country to be appropriately groomed and correctly married. She returned to the US triumphant and unmarried, picked up a passel of scholarships and completed a PhD. Tess has been a mother once, a wife twice, a waitress briefly and a college professor way too long. Her work as a writing consultant to corporate America continues to stimulate her mind and feed her body. Having swept away most of the encumbrances in her life, Tess now writes, paints, tends her beehives, plays with her grandchildren, travels, gardens and cooks on impulse and without ambition.

About the poem: "In 1972, my three-year-old son was recuperating from a mild case of chickenpox when his knee swelled up overnight. A staph infection diagnosis put him in the pediatric ward of a small-town hospital. What followed was weeks of uncertainty, continuous intravenous antibiotics, surgery, isolation and many tears. I was scolded for spending the first night on the floor next to his crib and for violating visiting-hour rules. My son's body healed, but his spirit was wounded: To this day, he cannot enter a hospital without feeling sick to his stomach. Pediatric wards are better now, of course, but no matter how brightly they're painted, it's a paucity of love and touch that leads to the cold desolation I tried to capture in this poem."

sweet lies

Marilyn Hillman
3/19/2010

I can sense the question before it comes.

"How are you doing?"

I want to answer, *How do you think I'm doing, with my husband morphing into a ghost? I'm dying here. But thanks for asking.*

Instead I clench my fists and deliver a cheerful response: "I'm good." Which is, of course, a lie.

My husband is demented.

I cannot say these words out loud. Pushed to the wall, I'll say that my husband has dementia, like it's temporary—a virus curable by bed rest and chicken soup. Murray admits only to memory problems, while I split hairs over which verb I can stand to put next to his decline. We skitter around the truth like insects caught in a pool of light and scurrying for cover. The reality is, we're on a steady downhill course, with Murray in frantic pursuit of words and ideas he can't remember, while I chase after him, trying to mine precious nuggets of coherence buried in his muddy ramblings.

Murray imagines himself still capable of living a richly layered life, despite what his psychiatrist calls a severely impaired executive function system. *What the hell is that?* I wonder. Like any medically illiterate person confronted with a diagnosis rendered in doctorspeak, I consult Wikipedia, where I learn that Murray can no longer plan or initiate appropriate actions, think abstractly or adapt to the unexpected.

Dementia has certainly demolished Murray's once formidable planning skills. "What am I doing today?" he asks me repeatedly. I answer each time, "Patrick is coming after breakfast." But when the physical therapist appears, my husband goes into shutdown. "What's he doing here?" Murray demands, as if I've backed him into a corner.

The irony stabs me in the gut. My brilliant husband, who once held the title Chairman, Marketing *Plans* Board at a global advertising firm, can no longer plan a single hour of his day.

Murray's losses are staggering. With his fragile and easily loosened grip on reality, he flits in and out of incoherent thought patterns, conflating unrelated ideas he picks up from CNN into bravely disjointed phrases brimming with meaningless content. "Aftershocks coming with the activities of that bird hiding behind a tire." This nonsense from a man who once prided himself on his razor-sharp intellect. I grieve for that unraveling intellect, for that gorgeous brain I found so compelling during our thirty-five years of marriage.

At eighty-seven, Murray has sixteen years on me, and maybe I should have expected our age difference to play out as it has. But who pictures the worst when you're young and crazy in love with a brainy, powerful man?

At times we're both guilty of indulging in the elaborate fiction that our life remains the same, unimpeded by the specter of mental deterioration hemming him in, closing off his options and constricting his autonomy. While Murray does not have Alzheimer's, his psychiatrist tells me that my husband is inexorably bound for the same black hole of oblivion. Instead of sliding quickly down the Alzheimer's slope, he'll make his way more slowly, with rest stops along the way, allowing him to retain whatever level of cognition he still has before the next drop-off.

I move to the beat of Murray's swings in mood and competence. Locked in a slow tango of deception and uncoupling, our cheeks pressed together, we sway to the rhythms of his disease. Murray takes a step backward into God knows where, and I follow, whispering my sweet lies: "Everything will be fine. You'll see, my darling." But even as I beguile him with untruths, I push myself forward into a life where he cannot join me, where I am alone with my fears, where I am in charge.

My husband, the former control freak, abdicated power with the most suc-cinct sentence: "You do it." Last year, when our basement was mysteriously filling with water, Murray flashed me his endearing smile and said, "You fix it." *Me? Hello?*

Yes, I now play the leading role in our family drama. Murray appears in an occasional cameo, taking out the trash or flooding the apartment with water he's forgotten to turn off, but mostly he prefers to nap or watch TV. I see him gradually withdrawing into his increasingly disheveled thoughts, leav-ing me to steer the ship.

Each day I say a silent goodbye to whatever has gone missing from his per-sonality. Memory, empathy and initiative have already peeled away, leaving a docile core neither of us would have believed possible.

Medicine has no magic bullet to fix my husband's dementia. At least not yet. And sadly, I will soon be living with an imposter, someone who no longer knows me or himself. I silently plead with God to give my husband a break, to let us coast for awhile, before his cognition disappears forever. As it will.

Farewell, my beloved husband. I will accompany you on your journey, but I cannot be your guide. You must find your way on that grim path alone. But not too soon, my sweet. Hang on. Dance with me just a little longer.

About the author: Marilyn Hillman is a photographer and writer. Her essays have appeared in The Healing Muse, The Yale Journal for Humanities in Medicine, Ars Medica *and* Epidemiology of Women's Health. *She began writing as a way to confront the realities of her husband's dementia and is currently working on a book about their journey through his illness.*

spring

Depression session

Abby Caplin
4/2/2010

The chopped apple of her father's eye,
She tastes the grapes of her mother's drunken wrath
The barely visible slivers of silver-tongued almond
Needle her intestines as she savors
The seedless watermelon of fruitless friendships,
And endures the hard rind
Of a body gone awry,
To be chewed and chewed until swallowed or
Spat out. A salad of sorts
Surrounded by lemons
Home-grown, organic, bitter
And full of juice. She brings me a tough
Clear plastic bag filled with them
To our session.
"They're the last of the season," she tells me.
I pray this is true,
While at home, I pore through cookbooks,
Searching for yet another recipe.

About the poet: Abby Caplin practices mind-body medicine in San Francisco, CA, counseling people with chronic illness.

About the poem: "When sitting with clients, I hold the space to hear about the psychological and physical wounds caused by illness and how challenges in their lives have impacted their health. The woman in this poem is a composite of people with whom I have worked, as well as a bit of myself. When a client brought me lemons from her tree and told me they were the last of the season, I was struck by the symbolism."

Babel: The voices of a medical trauma

Tricia Pil
4/9/2010

Editor's Note: On the eve of Pulse's *second anniversary, we offer a remarkable piece. It is the true story of a hospitalization as told from three points of view: first, the recollections of the patient (who happens to be a physician); second, events as recorded in the medical charts by doctors and nurses; and third, the version put forth by the hospital.*

FRIDAY

Patient:
It is fall 2005, and I am nine months pregnant. A healthy thirty-three-year-old pediatrician, I am a longtime patient of Doctor A and Doctor B, who delivered my two young children at this hospital. My husband and I are eagerly anticipating the birth of our third child.

One evening after dinner, the contractions start coming every five minutes. My husband and I pack our bags and drive to the hospital. I am nearly 4 cm dilated. After observation, Doctor C calls Doctor A, makes a diagnosis of false labor and sends us home.

Chart:
9:25 pm: 33 year old gravida 3, para 2, 38 5/7 week seen in office this AM almost 3 cm. Negative PMHx, c/o contractions q 5 min. Cervix 3+. Will ambulate 2 hours.

12:15 am: Continued contractions q 5 min. Spoke with Doctor A—home or stay—patient chooses to go home. Keep appointment Monday for induction.—Doctor C

Hospital:
Your presentation to Triage was discussed with Doctor A by the OB Triage Specialist. Since there was no change in cervical dilation, you were discharged.

SATURDAY

Patient:

My water breaks the following night, and I call Doctor B. After saying "Hold your horses," he grudgingly tells me to return to the hospital. By the time we arrive, my contractions are coming every minute. No one is behind the emergency room desk. My husband finally finds an off-duty orderly willing to get a wheelchair to take me to the birthing center. There, the secretary refuses to call a nurse until I sign papers explaining the hospital's privacy policies.

Chart:
Registration 10:45 pm Triage admission 10:45 pm

Hospital:
After 10:30 pm a call bell is present on the counter in case the triage nurse is not at the window. The "off duty orderly" who wheeled you upstairs to the birthing center may not have known the proper sequence to follow. Documented registration time is 10:45 pm and the time placed in the triage room is 10:45 pm which indicates swift placement into a triage room. There are some forms that must be signed for each admission.

Patient:

In triage, Doctor D prepares a fern test to determine whether the fluid that has soaked the bed and wheelchair has come from a ruptured amniotic sac, when that fact is clear even to my lay husband. Nurses are shouting at me not to push, but I am involuntarily bearing down with each contraction. By the time we rush towards the delivery room, the baby is crowning. He is born in the hallway.

Chart:
10:59 pm: Boy delivered 8 pounds, 1 ounce. Spontaneous vaginal delivery.—Nurse A

Hospital:
You delivered in the labor and delivery room 14 minutes after arrival by the OB Triage Specialist.

Patient:

I am left lying there, waiting for Doctor B. When he arrives I ask, "Where were you?" He answers, "I can't come until they call me." He yanks the placenta out, and I bite my lip. At one point, while he is sewing my laceration from the birth, I exclaim, "Ouch! I can feel that!" He replies, "Aww, that's just the deepest one," and keeps on going. He disappears as soon as he is done.

Chart:
11:25 pm: BP 136/76, HR 85. Hemoglobin 14.
Delivery Note: Precipitous labor, arrived at triage 8 cm, dilated and delivered on arrival by Doctor D. I arrived in room just after delivery. Placenta spontaneous and repair of second degree laceration under local. Group beta strep positive—no antibiotics given.—Doctor B

Hospital:
Doctor B was on-call for his practice that night and was physically on the premises. However, since your delivery progressed so quickly he did not make it from his prior location. He does not recall "yanking" your placenta.

SUNDAY

Patient:

We are moved to the postpartum floor. Seven hours later, I suddenly feel weak, dizzy and nauseated. I say, "Somebody help me, I don't feel well." The next minute, I'm hemorrhaging. There is blood spurting everywhere, clots the size of frying pans. I think I am going to die. Panicky nurses and residents crowd the room. The crash cart is wheeled in, my baby is wheeled out. My husband is shouting, "Somebody get Doctor B!" I am being stuck everywhere for an IV. Someone says that there will be a "procedure," and then my underwear is cut off, injections slammed into my buttocks, my legs are forced open and somebody shoves an entire forearm into my uterus and pulls out clots. Three times. I scream and scream and scream. The pain is unbearable, and I feel brutally violated.

Chart:
7:30 am: Called to see patient passing clots. Passed two medium size clots. Blood pressure 110/67…100/60…90/58. Pulse 88…96. Patient uncomfortable, vomited x 2. Bimanual evacuation lower uterine segment with 3 large clots. Orders: IV, Pitocin IV, Methergine IM, Morphine IM, Zofran prn. Discussed with Doctor B.—Intern

Hospital:
Once again, we refer you back to your private physician for a detailed discussion about the hemorrhage you outlined.

Patient:
Everyone flees the room.
I am curled in a fetal position, crying and shaking. No one comes to explain why, how or what has just happened. When my husband stumbles down the hall afterwards, other new mothers stop him to ask if his wife is okay after what they have heard. They are the only ones who ever ask if I am all right.

Chart:
7:40 am: BP 90/58. Will continue to observe.—Night Nurse B
8:00 am: IV running. Patient medicated with Zofran for nausea. Resting comfortably. Will monitor.—Day Nurse C

Hospital: [no response]

Patient:
Doctor B makes rounds. "You doctors make the worst patients." Then he asks if I am up for an early discharge. He stands in the doorway, making more eye contact with my chart than with me. I never see him again.

Chart:
8:40 am: Hemoglobin 11. BP 90/60.
Afebrile, vital signs stable. Fundus firm, lochia moderate, perineum ok. Doing well. Orders: Discontinue Pitocin at 12 noon if lochia normal. Heplock IV.—Doctor B

Hospital: [no response]

Patient:
My husband notices that the expiration date on the bag of Pitocin—the intravenous medication used to treat postpartum hemorrhage—is fourteen days overdue. A nurse quickly removes the bag and assures me that Pitocin is good for two weeks past its expiration date anyway.

Chart:
1:50 pm: IV infiltrate right forearm. Catheter discontinued.—Nurse D

Hospital:
Each unit where Pitocin is supplied is checked on a monthly basis. The Pitocin label has two dates on it. One date is the compound date, and the other is the expiration date. Is it possible you noticed the compound date?

Patient:
I lie dazed and in shock, unable to eat or drink. When my baby is brought in to nurse, I numbly put him to my breast and go through the motions. Patient-care assistants come in once per shift to chart my vital signs. Nurses avoid the room and act as if nothing happened.

Chart:
12 pm: BP 100/70. 4 pm: 90/60.
Intake: Regular diet. Quantity sufficient. Output: Voided. Quantity sufficient.
Infant weight 7 pounds, 10 ounces. Breastfeeding score 10/10. Assessment within normal limits.—Nursing notes

Hospital: [no response]

MONDAY

Patient:
Doctor A rounds. "I'm surprised you decided to leave that first night." I am stunned. When I finally answer that we were discharged from the emergency room on his orders, he replies, "I thought you came in looking for a sneak induction." He writes my discharge orders a day early and leaves, also never to be seen again.

Chart:
12 pm: BP 90/60. 8 pm: 96/58.
No complaints. Feeling better. Doing well breastfeeding. Orders: Home tomorrow AM.—Doctor A
Infant weight 7 pounds, 5 ounces.
Infant nursing well at frequent intervals. Exam significant for icterus [jaundice]…facial bruising…Precipitous delivery, maternal group beta strep positive without antibiotic treatment. Discharge planned for Day Five if course in hospital remains uneventful.— Doctor E

Hospital: [no response]

TUESDAY

Patient:
On the morning of discharge, I tell the nurses repeatedly that my baby is very sleepy, not nursing well and starting to vomit. He has lost 10 percent of his weight in the forty-eight hours since birth. The discharge nurse tells me to "stop worrying like a pediatrician mother," his vomit is just spit-up, and he is not sleepy, just "content." We are handed formula samples and hurried out the door.

Chart:
1:45 pm: Infant weight 7 pounds 3 ounces. Bilirubin 12.7. Report given to Doctor F via Nurse E. Patient discharged to home with infant after discharge instructions and supplemental nursing that patient requested

in case she decided to supplement infant. Patient's condition stable.—
Nurse F
MD verbal order: Discharge home with mother. Cancel home health.

Hospital:
There was no emesis or spitting documented. Status reports were given to Doctor F and nursing notes indicate that Doctor F wanted your baby to be supplemented. The nursing notes indicate that you were informed of this and were provided instruction on supplemental nursing.

Patient:
Within one hour of getting home, my baby throws up again, drenching the bassinet. We rush him to the pediatrician's office and are sent immediately to the emergency room of another hospital. He is jaundiced, lethargic and dehydrated. The ER staff struggles for IV access, sticking his arms, legs and scalp. He is admitted that evening, five hours after our hospital discharge, still wearing his hospital leg bands. It is my thirty-fourth birthday.

Chart:
6 pm: Infant weight 7 pounds, 3 ounces. Bilirubin 16.9. Sleepy, floppy, jaundice to umbilicus. Admit.—Emergency room notes

Hospital:
Once again your pediatrician can address your concern in this matter as well.

WEDNESDAY, THURSDAY, FRIDAY

Patient:
My son remains hospitalized, lying in an incubator receiving intravenous fluids and phototherapy. He doesn't come home for good until he is nearly a week old, requiring yet another week of home phototherapy and daily home-care visits before regaining his strength and weight.

Chart:
Diagnosis: Obstetrical Trauma Not Otherwise Specified.
Disposition: Return in approximately one year.—Doctor G

Hospital:
We are sorry that you were so unhappy with your stay. After a thorough investigation of your allegations, we have concluded that the care you received was appropriate. Thank you for taking the time to express your concerns.

In the months after my son's delivery, it was as if a curtain had descended over my life. In addition to a terrible feeling of numbness, I was haunted by flashbacks and nightmares about what had happened. Billboards for the hospital where I'd delivered, people dressed in scrubs, pregnant women, a favorite red velvet cake that now resembled to me a large blood clot and, worst of all, my own baby—the sight of any of these could trigger flashbacks and bouts of heart-stopping, sweat-drenched panic.

For my postpartum checkup, I saw a new obstetrician, who listened uncomfortably to my tearful story and ultimately dismissed my symptoms as hormone-induced baby blues, "Mother Nature's way of kicking women when they're down."

After five months of worsening symptoms, I finally self-referred to a psychologist who began treating me for post-traumatic stress disorder (PTSD). It was only then that I started bonding with my infant son.

On the eve of my son's first birthday, the first anniversary of the event, I wrote a letter of complaint to the hospital and to the physicians who'd been involved in our care. It had taken me that whole year to verbalize what had transpired. Even as I mailed the letter, I struggled with feelings of disbelief, anger, shame and betrayal that something like this could have happened to me, a physician, "one of their own."

I wrote the letter because I wanted the doctors and hospital staff to understand my perspective and to appreciate the devastating impact that this event had had on my life and family.

I also wanted them to consider the inept and unfeeling care we'd received from first to last—including the failure to get me into a delivery room quickly enough, the brutal response to the hemorrhage (which better care might have prevented in the first place) and the inappropriate discharge of my ill newborn.

I wanted them to change the way they conducted business so that no one else would have to endure what I did.

Naively enough, I wasn't even thinking of a lawsuit—that is, until I received the hospital's letter of reply three months later, the one extensively quoted above. In that infuriating moment I suddenly understood why patients sue. The response, with its defensive, denying, callous tone, was like a slap in the face—like being traumatized a second time.

The following week I called a malpractice lawyer and told him my story.

He listened sympathetically and then zeroed in on the key word—*damages*. Aside from my psychotherapy bills, it was hard to pinpoint a lasting physical injury to me or to my baby. "This case would be worth a lot more if we had three motherless children or a brain-dead baby in a wheelchair," he said. That's when I politely thanked him for his time.

I wanted an apology, answers and change—not money.

I never did receive a response from any of my physicians.

As someone who has been on the receiving end of care that felt both incompetent and uncaring, if not cruel, I'm sure that we medical professionals can do better. As someone who looked for explanations and received none, I'm hoping that we can change, getting beyond blame-shifting, defensiveness, denial and complicit silence—and moving instead towards transparency, disclosure, apology and healing.

As a physician, I hope that we can learn to more actively engage our patients in their own care. I hope that we can reexamine the ways in which we respond to our own errors and share the lessons we have learned with our medical students and residents.

If we can do this, perhaps then we could rise above the babble of Babel, our voices joined in a common language of human care and compassion.

———————————

About the author: *Before the events described above, Tricia Pil worked for six years as a pediatrician in private community practice. In the aftermath of the trauma, because of PTSD triggers present in the healthcare environment, she was for several years unable to return to clinical practice. She went back to college, rediscovered a love of writing and earned a second undergraduate degree in English literature. She is medical director of quality and safety at Children's Community Pediatrics in Pittsburgh and is once again a practicing pediatrician. She is dedicated to using her professional background as a pediatrician and her personal experience as a patient to advocate for improved quality and safety in health care and for increased awareness of postpartum PTSD.*

She wishes to thank James Conway, Jane Roessner PhD and Frank Davidoff MD at the Institute for Healthcare Improvement and Linda Kenney at Medically Induced Trauma Support Services for their steadfast encouragement and support. And she thanks Karen Katunich PhD "for saving my life."

The University Hospital of somewhere Else

Paula Lyons
4/16/2010

July 1. My first day as a family-medicine intern, assigned to Labor and Delivery, and my first night on call, 6 pm sharp. Enviously, I watched the other interns smartly packing up to go home.

"See you in the morning—maybe!" they joked.

I glanced at the status board: eight patients in labor. And now I was "in charge," at least in name, till 7 am report tomorrow.

Several chaotic hours later, I finished helping a Guatemalan mother of five to deliver her sixth son. My hands were trembling.

Toweling the plucky little newborn dry, I admitted the truth: Despite my University Hospital's proud reputation as a maternity center, this woman would probably have done as well or better in her own warm, clean, cilantro-scented kitchen. At best, I was superfluous; at worst, a comical hindrance.

In shaky Spanish I told her, *"Su hijo es muy guapo y tiene salud!"* (Your son is very handsome and healthy.)

"Lo se," she replied, smiling. *"Tranquila, doctorita. Todo estara bien."* (I know, little doctor. Be calm, all will be well.)

Washing my hands after the next "case" (a stoic Asian woman who gave birth silently and quickly), I glimpsed at my face in the mirror—cheeks drawn, lips pale and chapped. A far cry from how I'd looked at my wedding, just seventeen days earlier. I was already changing.

A page came from the postpartum floor, one flight down. I hurried downstairs to meet the charge nurse who'd paged me.

An Army-trained veteran, she sized me up, clearly recognizing a newbie, then gave me my orders: "YOU, get into room 8. The woman is sixteen years old, C-section this morning for breech twins, one died. She's hysterical and grieving. YOU go in there and calm her down."

An imposing Valkyrie, about my mother's age and twice her mass, she pointed imperiously at a door. Meekly, I went in.

I found my patient sitting in bed, braced bolt upright on her thin arms, and panting.

Something's off, my nascent doctor's brain muttered. She might be devastated, but something was off. That was a painful position for someone with a new abdominal incision....

And her face held a hint of gray. Well, she'd just had surgery—surely that was it?

She looked at me.

"Can't breathe," she puffed faintly.

Sticking to orders, I said, "I'm Dr. Lyons. This must be so terrible for you. Why don't you lie back, so we can talk?"

She let me ease her down into a reclining position, then snapped upright again.

"No! Can't breathe!"

I stared in horror. Everything came together in a rush: This wasn't hysteria, this was fluid! She was in pulmonary edema! Her lungs were full of fluid!

Panicked as I was, I never thought to confirm my diagnosis by listening to her heart or lungs, and I also forgot to start her on oxygen.

I ran to the nursing station.

"I need a syringe, a butterfly needle and heparin," I told the Valkyrie. "Where are they?"

She sighed, shook her head and showed me, gazing at me as if I were a new species of toad. The other nurses snickered.

As I drew the blood gas—a test to measure oxygen levels in the blood—from my patient's wrist, she never protested, just kept grimly panting. This frightened me even more, as arterial sticks really hurt.

The lab technician ran the specimen and handed me the paper strip with the oxygen reading: PO2= 54. Roughly half the right amount.

I emergency-paged the supervising resident. She yawned her reply over the phone: "You hit the vein." (Venous blood contains less oxygen than arterial blood.)

"Why didn't you call the Arterial Stick Team?" she continued. "Have them re-draw her blood."

Chastened, I hung up. But I was certain I'd been in the artery: I'd seen the blood pump, pump, pump its way up the tubing. (Arterial blood pumps; venous blood doesn't.)

The Art Stick Team appeared, repeated the procedure and took the specimen to the lab.

Waiting for the test results, I sat on the bed with my patient and gently rubbed her straining back. As her thin torso welled and sank painfully, I told her, "Don't worry, it's okay, you're going to be fine."

I tried to sound resolute, but my cheeks blazed with fear, uncertainty and humiliation. Maybe I was wrong—maybe this was grief after all. Or maybe my patient was in real trouble. What a way to begin my internship! What the hell ever made me think I could do this job?

Suddenly the room filled with people—nurses, residents, techs, medical assistants, even the attending physician! I was shoved out of the way, and they administered oxygen, inserted IVs and converted my "crashing" patient (likely to die without fast help) into an ICU case.

As they whisked my patient away in a stretcher, the second-year resident flung back at me: "Postpartum cardiomyopathy, or maybe a PE." (Postpartum heart failure, or maybe a blood clot to the lungs.)

My patient's glassy eyes met mine fleetingly. I had just enough time to feel how I'd failed her. Then she was gone.

Shaken and drained, I walked back to the nurses' station and flopped down heavily into a chair.

Mentally I reviewed my performance. Christ! I'd done so many things wrong! Didn't examine my patient thoroughly, didn't start oxygen, drew the art stick myself....

Worst of all, I'd come this close to treating this young woman as "just" a grieving teenage mother. If she died, would it be my fault?

I thought of her surviving baby, curled up in the NICU. I thought of my brand-new husband, sleeping peacefully in our tiny home, and wrenched back confused tears.

I noted the time: 4:27 am. Twelve more hours of call to go. Letting my head fall into my hands, I tried to brace myself.

Suddenly there was a figure at my elbow, and a booming voice.

"Here, Doctor, I thought you might like this."

A steaming, fragrant cup of coffee appeared beside me. Startled, I looked up into the Valkyrie's eyes—now guardedly approving.

"Huh? Oh! Wow, thank you very much," I said. "This smells great."

She smiled briefly and turned away. As I sipped the life-giving elixir, I realized that I'd passed some kind of test. She clearly held no grudge. In a scant, terrifying half-hour, I had gone from being "YOU" to being "Doctor."

My pager buzzed: Labor and Delivery. God only knew what was happening up there. I grabbed another quick sip of my scalding coffee and bolted for the stairs.

About the author: Paula Lyons is a native of New Jersey who graduated from Emory University School of Medicine. She now practices family medicine just outside of Baltimore, MD. Some of her other writings have appeared in Pulse, The Pharos *and* The Journal of Family Practice.

Triptych for John

Yun Lan
4/23/2010

Part I: The first time I saw you

I met John
without
John,
without introduction.
Cold,
cold,
cold hand.

Part II: Cadaver as Decapod

John was surely a hermit crab, having four small limbs to anchor the body and six long limbs to advance it. He gathered sea anemones on his back, and weeds in his spiny beard. He bore stellate scars, the digitated marks of five pointed teeth. There was a constellation of them, surely from the care of blue spined urchins. The urchins couldn't make him stay. Did they evict him or had he just outgrown his home?

Surely, his soft belly was turned out to the brine, the ocean full of predators. In each eye of many lenses, what did he see? Was he afraid to scuttle from this white ribbed shell to the larger? Perhaps not. He trusted he could replace his old limbs. He could carry anemones to protect him. He would fear neither octopus, nor fellow crabs, nor stars.

We can pick at the questions, we each with ten limbs: sharp scissors, blunt scissors, olive point probe, teasing wooden handled straight needle, thumb forceps, "fitted teeth" tissue forceps with 1x2 jaws, Jones artery forceps, straight eye forceps, stout probe, and scalpel. Trace his spiral atria. Study the attachments—how his limbs clung to this concavity. Then, saw from sinus through concha, and chisel to where his eyes hid. We know just the angle and just the force to pince the bone.

We are surely young hermit crabs, still small enough to make John's shell our new home.

Part III: Ode to the Donor

My practiced nonchalance at pulling
fat from skin could not prepare me for
the treasures that I found within:

a perfect ruby—the size of a pea, a piano,
its thousand strings, and worn
white lacquer keys.

Beside a river was a crane bowed low against the dawn,
to welcome every cargo load,
to lift on and on and on.

Volumes of voice and discipline were written in his flesh.
Could I study only
syllables, their pathways and their breadth?

What is the body's story?
A machine at its best? A way to know hunger,
and sickness and death?

I ask this remnant
of a face. I wait
and watch your lips.

I ask, what is a body? You say,
It is
a gift.

When time for giving
time was gone, still you gave again.
Was it to cease the ceasing, or yield to end as end?

May I too give beyond to heal the hurt and bruised.
It is my only way to say,
"John, thank you.

Thank you."

About the poet: *Yun Lan (a pen name) is a medical student.*

About the poem: *"I wanted to describe phases in my experience of anatomy lab. I also wanted to write a piece to share with classmates and faculty at our ceremony to honor those whose remains we've dissected."*

Making Headlines

Reeta Mani
4/30/2010

"Did he die of swine flu?" demanded a scrawny man wearing a blue shirt and green surgical mask. He was one of a throng of news reporters packing the lobby of a private hospital in the heart of Bangalore, my city.

It was early August 2009, and India had just recorded its first casualty from the novel H1N1 influenza virus. This latest variant of influenza—a chimera of swine, avian and human flu genes—was raising grave concerns among the medical community worldwide. To try to contain a pandemic, countries were ordering stockpiles of antiviral drugs and initiating vaccine production on a wartime footing.

In Bangalore, as elsewhere, you could pick up any newspaper or watch any news channel and see headlines screaming "Swine Flu!" Men, women and children wore masks of all sizes, shapes and hues. Paranoia was at its peak: An innocuous sneeze could make people run helter-skelter for cover.

A few H1N1 cases had been confirmed in Bangalore, but fortunately none had been fatal. The local media, on the alert 24–7, were hounding any doctor associated with the diagnosis or treatment of swine flu. If word went out that a local hospital had a suspected case of swine flu, the press descended in swarms.

At this hospital, a seventeen-year-old boy who'd been admitted with a serious lung infection the previous day had died in the early hours of the morning. Somehow reporters had gotten wind of it—and so here they were, masks on, waiting for the boy's doctor to come out and make an announcement.

They were clearly hoping for a scoop: "City's first swine flu death!"

Although I was part of the H1N1 diagnostic testing team from the city's public virology laboratory, I was here on personal business—meeting a colleague so that we could visit a mutual acquaintance who'd been admitted to the hospital for an acute asthma attack. Waiting in the lobby, I watched the reporters gather.

And then they grew restless: To go to press they needed to hear the doctor in charge confirm that the boy had died of swine flu. When they realized that some of the deceased boy's relatives were right there waiting as well, they began firing questions:

"Did the doctors tell you he had swine flu?"

"Was he tested for swine flu?"

"When did his symptoms start?"

"Did anyone else in the family have the same symptoms?"

The relatives, overwhelmed by the boy's death, were too agonized to speak. But I could sense their anger, pain and frustration at the reporters' insensitive, incessant questions, and at the delay in being able to receive their loved one's remains. (As per protocol in India, hospital authorities hand over the deceased's body to relatives, who take it home so that family members and friends can pay last respects and complete traditional rituals before the body is cremated.) For a moment I worried that the relatives might run out of patience and explode under the reporters' barrage.

"Leave the family alone!" I wanted to shout. But there were so many reporters; I felt too puny to take them on. Besides, letting them know that I was in any way associated with swine flu would be catastrophic. I would become a new target for their unwanted attentions—and I wasn't even an employee of this hospital.

Shut up, I decided, and let the deceased boy's physician do the talking.

Finally he appeared. A hush descended, the air thick with suspense and anticipation.

The boy had died of a lung infection, the doctor confirmed. Then he added, "But he tested negative for swine flu. He died of pulmonary tuberculosis."

I expected the reporters to pounce upon him, demanding more information and clarifications. Instead, I heard only disappointed murmurs and sighs. Then they dispersed, pulling off their masks. They'd lost their scoop.

The news of the young man's death from tuberculosis didn't make it into any newspaper.

Why would it? In India, tuberculosis kills two people every three minutes. Each year my country sees about 1.9 million new cases, roughly half of them "open"—that is, infectious to others like this unfortunate, once healthy seventeen-year-old.

A deadly disease.

But too ancient and common to be newsworthy.

About the author: Reeta Mani is a virologist at the National Institute of Mental Health and Neurosciences (NIMHANS) in Bangalore, India. "Since childhood I have always loved to write. My profession earns me my bread and butter, but as a writer I have the freedom to express what I cannot possibly as a doctor. I write to free myself of thoughts that plague me, issues that dishearten me and inequities that leave me feeling helpless."

Ladies in waiting

Alan Blum
5/7/2010

Editor's Note: This week, Pulse *ventures into new territory. We present sketches by a family physician who for years has been jotting down visual impressions and snippets of conversation as he cares for patients. These sketches go back as far as thirty-five years, representing patients who have died or with whom he lost touch because of geographic relocation. These drawings were first published in* Ladies in Waiting, *a letterpress printed book, in one edition of seventy-five copies.*

About the author: *Alan Blum MD (ablum@cchs.ua.edu) is professor and endowed chair in family medicine at the University of Alabama, Tuscaloosa, where he also directs the Center for the Study of Tobacco and Society. In 1977 he co-founded DOC (Doctors Ought to Care), the first international physicians' anti-smoking organization. For his contributions to health promotion, Dr. Blum received the Surgeon General's Medallion from Dr. C. Everett Koop and an honorary Doctor of Science by Amherst College. His sketches and stories of patients have appeared in numerous publications, including* Literature and Medicine, The Pharos, JAMA *and* Canadian Medical Association Journal.

About the sketches: *"These sketches were all unplanned and were done with ballpoint pen on whatever paper I happened to have in my hand at the time, from prescription pads and paper towels to the wrappers of latex gloves or sterile gauze. As a medical student at Emory, I began adding sketches to my notes as a way to spend a bit more time with the patient, to focus more closely on the patient's expression and to try to capture the essence of our encounter. I learned the importance of listening closely to patients from my father, a general practitioner in Queens, New York. His office was in our home, where every afternoon the living room became the waiting room. A central role of a personal physician is to identify the patient's fears and to try to allay anxiety. There's a patient in all of us, waiting to get out.*

I don't see why they have to have
all those syllables
just to say one word.
I like older doctors.
They seem to talk to you more.
Just like you talkin'.
Younger doctors seem to be in such a hurry.
I had one doctor,
used to have to chase him,
grab onto his white coat.
Flittin' up and down the hall.
You want to ask him somethin'
you have to run him down.

they have good cat fish for lunch?
yes but it
don't bodder me
he just fell in love i me

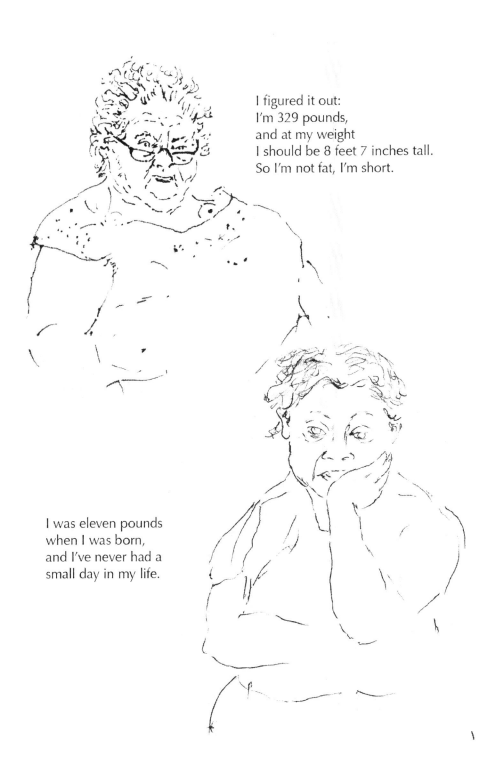

I figured it out:
I'm 329 pounds,
and at my weight
I should be 8 feet 7 inches tall.
So I'm not fat, I'm short.

I was eleven pounds
when I was born,
and I've never had a
small day in my life.

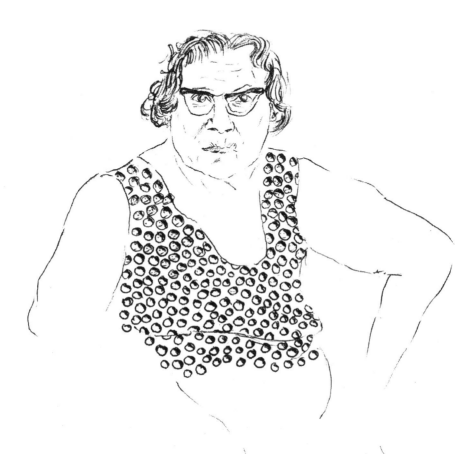

I had a hysterectomy.
It was done just before the Challenger blew up.
I have a tendency to remember dates.
I gave up smoking on Valentine's Day.
I gave up drinking on Thanksgiving.
Maybe it's because they dropped the atomic bomb on Hiroshima
on my second birthday.

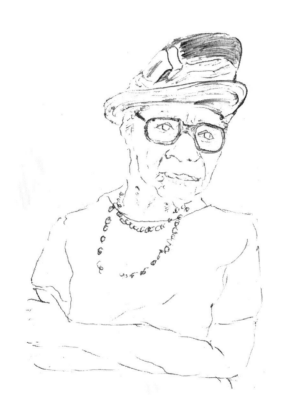

That doctor I saw
didn't know anything about polio.
Said it just weren't her generation
to know anything about it.
I can't remember that doctor's name,
as many bills as I got from her.

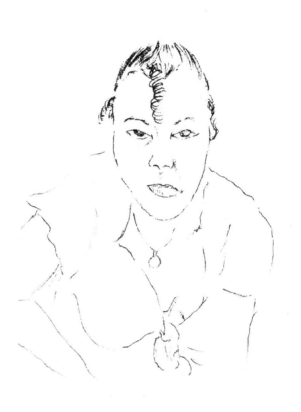

I came in early today
because I had this weird psychic feeling
you were running on time.

The Disabled Boat

Steve Gunther-Murphy
5/14/2010

Drifting on the sea of disease
in a cardboard boat,

never knowing when the slash
of a spinal eel
will lunge from its coral-bone cave
and cut through
the threads
of a once dancing ankle
or the push of a thigh
singing race or run.

Waiting without wanting—
as the slap of a wave
against the paper-thin stern
then bow
brings on the storm
that pummels every movement
until you slip into a coma of the wind;

your sails ripped from the mainstay
and the tar between the rails
yelling like the death of a two-year-old child.

You wake weeks
later
and notice
that your keel is gone;

your body shakes like a rock cod against
the pith of the boat's floor
with the hook deep in your gill;
making you talk in slow motion
and without air.

Who wants to live this life
of a shadow fish,
pulled from the depths of who you were
and gutted of simple motions
or the ability to sing glee from your gullet?

This is not the space I am.

This is not the blue snap of yesterday
that burst forth from my mother's womb
like an iris
on an island of moss rock.

About the poet: Steve Gunther-Murphy works in IT Healthcare at Kaiser Permanente in Oakland, California. He's been writing poetry since the seventh grade, has had works published in a variety of magazines and poetry journals and has given poetry readings in Hawaii, Colorado and California. "The muse tends to find me at all hours of the day and night and in all locations, so I have carried a poetry journal with me for over thirty years. I'm married, with two daughters. One is in her second year of veterinary school at UC Davis; the other works for a Boston healthcare nonprofit. My wife is a marriage and family therapist. Among the four of us, we engage some part of the earth's, animals' and human beings' health, inside and out."

About the poem: "Some time ago, an unusual heart virus forced me to stop my regular activities—biking, hiking, surfing, gardening and even basic housekeeping—for more than a year. All I could do besides my day-to-day work was to rest, eat and sleep. I fell into a dark well. While I was there, this poem rose to the surface. And when I came back, I realized that I wanted to dedicate the poem to two friends. One is Teresa Harris, a former athletic star who was disabled in her prime by debilitating arthritis and fibromyalgia and who inspires me by nonetheless letting the sunlight deep in her heart shine through her life. The other friend is Ellen Case, an avid and energetic bike rider who was struck by multiple sclerosis and yet still manages to grow garden flowers inside and outside and to keep going."

Adverse Effects

Kenny Lin
5/21/2010

Flashback to summer of 2008. I'm looking forward to August 5—the day that I'll no longer be a faceless bureaucrat. The day that the US Preventive Services Task Force (USPSTF) will issue its new recommendations on screening for prostate cancer—recommendations I've labored on as a federal employee for the past year and a half.

For much of 2007 I combed the medical literature for every study I could find on the benefits and harms of prostate cancer screening. In November of that year I presented my findings to the USPSTF, a widely respected, independent panel of primary-care experts They discussed and debated what the evidence showed and then voted unanimously to draft new recommendations. I didn't get to vote, but it has been my job in 2008 to shepherd the draft statement and literature review through an intensive vetting process and to finalize both.

As August 5 approaches, my colleagues in public relations warn me that the last time the USPSTF said anything about prostate cancer screening, the phones started ringing off the hook. I'm not so secretly hoping that the same will happen this time.

And I'm not disappointed! After we release the statement, my normally placid government agency buzzes with excitement. In addition to sparking front-page stories in major national newspapers, the story brings our PR office "hits" from television, internet and radio outlets all over the country. With the volume of requests far exceeding what the Task Force's press-liaison person can handle, I offer to pitch in. I give two newspaper interviews and debate a respected urologist on a live radio call-in show. My colleagues cheer me on. I forward the radio clip to my friends and family.

The new recommendations surprise many people: They say that men age seventy-five and older should not be screened for prostate cancer.

Why not?

Because there's no convincing proof that the prostate-specific antigen (PSA) blood test—the one used to detect early prostate cancer—actually saves lives. Most abnormal PSA tests do not actually indicate cancer, and up to half of true prostate cancers detected with the test would never have caused health problems if they'd gone undetected.

On the other hand, there's lots of evidence that the PSA test causes physical and psychological damage. Abnormal tests lead to prostate biopsies, operations and other treatments whose adverse effects range from anxiety to surgical complications to death. For younger men with decades of life remaining, these adverse effects may be worth the potential benefits; in men aged seventy-five and older, they almost certainly are not.

I soon learn that cancer recommendations, like cancer screening tests, come with their own adverse effects.

Comments pour into health blogs and the editorial pages of my favorite newspapers, accusing the Task Force, and me personally, of "ageism" and "taking the first step toward government-sponsored euthanasia." The systematic review I worked so hard on is trashed as a "shoddy meta-analysis" (although it's neither shoddy nor a meta-analysis), and many elderly men and their spouses lambaste us for being in league with heartless insurance companies.

I realize that this report has hit a nerve—the one that distrusts the health-care system and that lacks faith in government. Cancer inspires more fear and anxiety than many other diseases. People worry about being denied access to cancer care—even care that hurts more than it helps.

I'm most wounded by one comment, which says that those responsible for developing the guideline can't possibly understand what it's like to have, or to care for someone with, prostate cancer.

This one really pains me because I do understand.

I remember only too well a seventy-five-year-old patient—I'll call him Kendall—whom I met during my residency training in Lancaster, Pennsylvania, an area best known as Amish country. Kendall wasn't Amish, yet he hadn't seen a doctor in decades. Before I met Kendall, he'd been hospitalized with bone pain and a PSA of over 5000 (more than 4 is considered suspicious) and had been diagnosed with advanced, metastatic prostate cancer.

Kendall responded dramatically to a course of hormone-deprivation therapy and returned home. As I learned over the course of our outpatient visits, he was a man of few words but big gestures. At the end of our time together, he'd stand and clasp my right hand tightly in both of his, saying, "See you in a few months, doc."

Later, when the cancer and its awful pain returned, and Kendall became weaker, he was one of my favorite home-visit patients.

The end came surprisingly quickly. A hospice nurse paged me with the news that Kendall was in the ER, disoriented and combative. I rushed over and tried to soothe him as we ran tests, hoping in vain to find something we could fix. Soon afterwards, he was transferred to an inpatient hospice. He died a few days later.

Would PSA testing and earlier detection have spared or prolonged Kendall's life? Given the aggressiveness of his cancer, I doubt it, but it's hard to know for sure. And I admit that Kendall often came to mind as I was working on a recommendation to stop PSA testing at age seventy-five. If he'd ever bothered to visit a doctor, maybe he would have been one of the few men helped by such testing, rather than one of the many harmed. I'll never know.

My colleagues and I labored for months to present a thorough and accurate review that would help the USPSTF make sensible recommendations aimed at doing the most good and the least harm. We performed our work without considering healthcare costs or political fallout.

I'd hoped that August 5 would free me from being labeled a faceless bureaucrat. Ironically, it ended up tarring me as a heartless one.

Prostate cancer causes a lot of suffering—I know. In the face of that, it's tempting to try and detect it early, to "do something." But for now, unfortunately, our best science tells us that doing something to a man older than seventy-five is likely to do more harm than good.

For Kendall's sake and for my own—for I hope to be seventy-five myself one day—I wish it weren't that way.

I wish that on August 5, 2008, I'd had better news to share.

And I wish that everyone had understood that.

––––––––––––––

About the author: *Kenny Lin is associate deputy editor for the journal* American Family Physician *and director of the primary-care health fellowship at Georgetown University School of Medicine. Previously a medical officer for the US Preventive Services Task Force program at the Agency for Healthcare Research and Quality, he is also a former blogger for* US News & World Report. *Since July 2009, Dr. Lin has regularly shared his views on health and health-policy topics on his blog,* Common Sense Family Doctor (commonsensemd. blogspot.com).

pearls before swine

Kate Peters
5/28/2010

I'm a third-year medical student, and I'm starting the second day of my new rotation—a month that I'll spend with a family physician, Dr. Bauer, in his small, efficient home-based office.

Yesterday, my first day, a young woman named Sara came in for "strep throat." She had dark Latina eyes, broad cheekbones and a delicate tattoo of the Chinese character for "dream" on her left wrist. She was seventeen and seeking out a primary-care doctor for the first time in her life; I applauded her for taking responsibility for her own health care. Her tonsils were big and purple, covered in pus, but the rapid strep test was negative. She also reported a vaginal discharge. Dr. Bauer wanted to do a pelvic exam to check for a sexually transmitted disease (STD). He started her on antibiotics, ordered some blood tests and told her to return today to discuss her lab results and have the pelvic exam.

Now Sara returns with her mother, wanting to know why the exam was scheduled. Impressed by Sara's thoughtfulness, I tell her that we recommend the test, but assure her that the choice is hers. She looks me in the eye, confidently reports no STD risk and decides to wait on the pelvic exam.

Minutes later, I hear voices rising. Dr. Bauer seems to be, well, having a temper tantrum.

"You came here because I'm a doctor! Do you want to be treated by a doctor or not? I went to medical school! What do *you* know?"

Sara and her mother try to respond, but don't get more than a word out before he interrupts. It's not even an argument, really, because Dr. Bauer isn't listening or reasoning with them at all. His words and tone are insulting, arrogant and belittling.

Sara storms out of the office. Her mother stays behind to argue with the receptionist (who happens to be Dr. Bauer's wife), banging a pen into the counter, threatening to report the doctor's behavior. After they're gone, Dr. Bauer remains furious, and though Mrs. Bauer has been supporting him and helping him document the incident, he yells at her also.

I step out of the office, pace the parking lot and say a little prayer for composure.

I don't understand what has happened, or what could justify Dr. Bauer's reaction. I hate to hear people demeaning one another. If I heard a stranger on the street speaking to someone the way Dr. Bauer spoke to Sara, I'd probably intervene. But my position as a student, new to this rotation, doesn't seem to allow me that luxury. It's as if I can't be myself.

I fume behind my book for the rest of the day. I can't look Dr. Bauer in the eye. Throughout the afternoon he and Mrs. Bauer spin the story over and over.

"She just a slut and doesn't want anyone to know it!" Dr. Bauer hisses.

"And her ignorant spic mother doesn't even care," his wife adds loudly.

My face is hot with anger. Their language is not only bigoted, judgmental and mean, it's also deeply offensive to my personal beliefs.

"You see how God winnows them out for us?" Dr. Bauer says, wagging his finger, flaring his nostrils and hiking up his belt like he's ready for a fight. "The Lord didn't allow that awful patient to be in our practice! Cast not your pearls before swine!"

I feel myself physically cringe.

Dr. Bauer's little office is plastered with Christian pamphlets and Bible verses that his children have crayoned onto printer paper. His car has a Jesus license-plate placard and a little crucifix air freshener hanging from its rear-view mirror. This is a culture with which I'm well-acquainted; for many years, it was mine.

Though my evolving beliefs are nontraditional, I'm still rather enamored of the person of Jesus. I deeply believe that if God exists, then he or she is reflected in acts of love, compassion, justice, creativity, beauty, generosity. I feel outraged that Dr. Bauer would call his own bold unkindness and disrespect of another human being an act of God.

And yet I remain silent. I feel gagged by my position as a student, a subordinate. So at the end of the day I'm disgusted both with Dr. Bauer and with myself, driving out-of-state plates too fast down a country road.

I take a deep breath, coast, downshift. After a few minutes I call my friend who is a resident. He lets me vent a little, and finally I ask his advice.

"Your job is basically to agree for two years," he tells me. "You just have to play the game and learn what you can."

Really? Dr. Bauer didn't breach medical duty, but he did break other rules: He thwarted and denigrated Sara's attempts to make her own medical decisions and to use the healthcare system responsibly. Is this reportable? Do I have any recourse?

The phrase "First, do no harm" resonates in my mind. Doesn't being judgmental, arrogant and verbally abusive count as harm?

Three years ago, a group of professionals decided that I belong in the medical community. They accepted me because they saw my potential to become a healer, and in doing so, they made a promise to teach me how. But now one of my teachers is acting cruelly. How do I refuse his example but still remain his student? And can I still somehow be a healer to Dr. Bauer's patients?

Maybe I should call my school administration and ask to be removed from this rotation, at risk of falling behind by a couple of precious weeks; maybe I should notify the board of medicine.

After a long walk I sit down with trusted friends and rehash my conflicted day. They nod like sages and quietly suggest, "Well, maybe Dr. Bauer can still teach you something." As I open my mouth to disagree, they add, "And maybe he needs you to teach him something as well."

In the end, I decide to stay.

I'll learn what I can from Dr. Bauer and let go of the rest. But I'll also hold onto my beliefs, question what I'm told and see if I can't find a way to be honest and be myself.

There needs to be room for that in medical education—even in Dr. Bauer's tiny office.

––––––––––

About the author: Kate Peters wrote this story while in medical school. Now she continues to enjoy people and listen to stories while learning full-spectrum family medicine at the Ventura Family Medicine Residency in California, amid endlessly supportive and compassionate teachers. She is profoundly grateful and fulfilled in her vocation as a physician, but also eagerly awaits seasons of more free time to pursue other loves, including family and writing.

grandmother

Elizabeth Kao
6/4/2010

Today, her head is spinning, just like yesterday,
And the day before that. She is dizzy, experiencing
pain we can't know unless our heads have hurt like
she hurts now. All she wants is to lie down, and
when we tell her she just woke up, she says she
can't sleep, because we don't understand that
she's not concerned with the sleeping. She's the
same with food, telling us everything tastes bad,
merely eating to keep from being hungry.

She felt nothing to be worth doing after the fence fell,
just another part of a neglected house, but not
so neglected as to scream injustice to the world.
No one would mind that she did nothing, nor
would she—or more accurately, she didn't care.
So she turned inward, after seventy-three years of
War, raising a daughter and two sons, watching the
grandchildren for them, then left alone because
she seemed strong, for their convenience.

Tomorrow she will get up, eat breakfast, and sit
in her chair. By the afternoon, she will lie down in
her bed again, staring into space, wishing the pain
but not-pain will go away. And we blame a
chemical imbalance and wonder whether we should
have brought her to live with us, or put her in
another home, but ultimately decide that we can't
do much without affecting the normality of our lives,
what people will say, the time we have to give.

And I wonder whether I should hope for her to ever
get better, to be the grandmother who will tell
stories of life in Shandong, who will sing
and will show me jump-roping tricks.
I'm afraid to hope for things
that may not happen.

I ask if I don't care
or can't care,
or will care.

About the poet: Elizabeth Kao is a third-year medical student at the University of Oklahoma College of Medicine. She graduated in 2010 from Stanford University, where this poem was written with the encouragement of Dr. Larry Zaroff through the course Novels and Theater of Illness.

About the poem: This poem reflects upon depression and a grandchild's wish that she and her family could appreciate and care for her grandmother more.

ms. taylor

Remya Tharackal Ravindran
6/11/2010

Ms. Taylor was one of three newly hospitalized patients I saw that morning. She was a previously healthy woman in her forties, single and childless, who worked in the fashion industry. As I scanned her admission notes, three things stood out: shortness of breath, elevated calcium level and kidney failure. I read on, thinking of possible causes, then something caught my eye. Her breast exam had revealed multiple breast masses, and her chest x-ray showed fluid-filled lungs.

Everything fell into place: cancer, first in the breast and then spreading to the lungs. I was spared a diagnostic challenge, but I now had to face something more difficult—talking with Ms. Taylor about her diagnosis. Did she even know what it was? It didn't seem so.

For me, breaking bad news is an elusive art. As I walked to Ms. Taylor's room, I tried to recollect some of the strategies I'd been taught, like finding out what the patient thinks is going on and asking how much he or she wants to know. Still, I didn't know how Ms. Taylor would react. I felt nervous.

Ms. Taylor was sitting upright in bed, wearing an oxygen tube. She was a thin woman; the unkempt strands of silver hair falling over her pale, hollow cheeks made her look older than her years.

"Good morning!" she said, smiling. "Are you next in line to examine my breasts?" As frail as she seemed, she also radiated unmistakable spirit.

During the interview, I learned that breast cancer runs in her family. And when I examined her, I had no trouble finding the masses—reddish, peanut-sized lumps in both breasts, clearly visible and disturbingly hard.

Yet Ms. Taylor seemed nonchalant.

"Oh, I've had these since my teenage years," she said casually. "They would come and go; I've never paid much attention to them."

"Ms. Taylor, what do you think is going on with you?" I asked.

"The other doctor told me that I would need a biopsy to find out," she replied.

"What do you think the biopsy will show?" I persisted.

She shrugged and gave me a quizzical smile, eyebrows raised. Then she looked away and fixed her gaze on the window. Outside, a beautiful sunrise was in progress, the New York skyline perched on the distant horizon.

Kübler-Ross's stages of grief flashed through my mind. Which of them was Ms. Taylor experiencing—denial or acceptance? I couldn't quite tell. But it was obvious that she needed some time to herself. And I wasn't sure whether anything I could say would help her come to grips with the catastrophic news looming ahead. I said good day and silently retreated, letting her snuggle into her own thoughts.

When I saw Ms. Taylor again, a couple of days later, she no longer wore the oxygen tube. At my suggestion, the thoracic surgeon had inserted a needle between two ribs and drained five liters of fluid from the space surrounding her lungs.

"Breathing hasn't felt this good in a long time," Ms. Taylor told me.

I in turn breathed a sigh of relief: My suggestion hadn't been futile. My feelings of inadequacy at not being able to help her gave way to a sense of accomplishment.

For a few days, we continued Ms. Taylor's care—managing her fluid intake, adjusting her pain medications—while awaiting her biopsy results. I was midway through my internship, spending long hours at the hospital and feeling guilty for not spending more time with my four-year-old daughter. Meanwhile, my husband seemed at risk of losing his job. At moments, my own life seemed precarious, making me feel overwhelmed and helpless.

When Ms. Taylor's biopsy results arrived, they revealed invasive carcinoma. And her bone scan showed widespread bone metastases.

Though I knew that she'd already talked about her diagnosis with the oncologist, the thought of facing Ms. Taylor made me queasy. What did I have to offer her beyond kind words and more fluids? Filled with misgivings, I walked into her room.

She seemed too calm and collected for someone who had just received such grave news. In one hand was a prayer book.

"Doctor Wilson told me everything," she said flatly.

"Ms. Taylor..." I began.

"Do you believe in God?" she interrupted.

"Yes, I do," I replied. Though I was born into a Hindu family, I believe in one universal spirit. I have always found solace and strength in Hindu, Buddhist and Christian scriptures. I believe that the soul, like the body, needs to be fed and nourished every day.

"Good for you," she said, her eyes glittering with unshed tears. We gazed at each other in silence.

It occurred to me that Ms. Taylor had reached a sense of acceptance. Now, her nonchalance had the feeling of the calm after a storm. Even her interruption, I felt, was a skillful way of saving me from offering awkward, empty words of comfort. And "Good for you" was her way of reassuring me that I would be all right—and so would she.

She smiled at me. "The real stuff is so unlike *Grey's Anatomy*."

Though I didn't know much about the show, I appreciated her touch of humor. We chatted for a while longer—not about her illness but about her job, her church and the book of biblical excerpts she was reading.

Closing Ms. Taylor's door behind me, I felt a pang. As she faced her own death, Ms. Taylor had taught me something about life—at a time when my own life was filled with stress and uncertainty.

I will always remember her for her ability to appreciate and be grateful for the fragile and fleeting "now," even under such terrifying circumstances.

———————————

About the author: Remya Tharackal Ravindran has completed her residency at Overlook Hospital, Summit, NJ, and is currently doing a geriatrics fellowship at Baystate Medical Center, Springfield, MA. She grew up in India where she did her MBBS (the equivalent of an MD) in Trivandrum Medical College, Kerala. After graduation, she came to the US with her husband, who is an engineer, and their daughter. "This is my very first story, except for one published case report. I haven't written much since my high school days. My hobbies (although I hardly have time for them anymore) include astrology, reading scriptures, philosophy, painting and cooking."

stuck

Ken Gordon
6/18/10

I have never told this story to anyone.

It all started one night about ten years ago, three months into my internship. I was on call, having just admitted a man with a possible meningitis.

He now lay curled up in fetal position on the bed in front of me, looking thin and ill. Preparing to administer a lumbar puncture (a diagnostic test that involves removing fluid from the spinal canal), I gently pushed his head further down towards his legs.

He told me that he knew he was dying. AIDS had been ravaging his body for years. He wondered aloud whether this was a punishment for his previous lifestyle—especially the drugs. Everyone he'd cared for had either died or left him.

As I listened, I placed the spinal needle into the curvature of his back. I thought about dignity—something he hadn't experienced much of in the last few years. He seemed so close to death; I wondered briefly whether making a diagnosis of meningitis would be of any real help to him—whether we had anything to offer him in the last stages of this terrible disease. Then I thrust the needle into his spinal column.

I used too much force. The patient jerked, waking me from my reverie and bouncing the needle out of my right hand and into my left index finger. Then the needle dropped to the floor.

"Shit!" Running to the bathroom, I swiftly inspected the small puncture wound in my glove, then tore it off and glared at my finger. No blood! Was that good or bad? How deep was the puncture? Did I feel any pain? I quickly turned on the hot water and vigorously scrubbed my hand with soap.

I dried my hands. It was 3 am, and I felt tired and afraid. I knew that there was a hospital protocol for dealing with needlesticks—but feeling alone in a new city, without a soul to confide in, I panicked.

Instead of calling my senior resident for help, I did what seemed the easiest thing: I walked back to the patient, finished his lumbar puncture and didn't tell anyone what had happened.

I also did my best not to think about it again. When it did cross my mind, I felt terrified. What if I developed AIDS and died? What if getting a finger-stick so early in my internship meant that I was incompetent—that I would never be a good physician? I pushed these thoughts aside.

Shortly after this incident, the patient died from complications of crypto-coccal meningitis. He died alone. We were unable to locate any next-of-kin.

* * * * *

About a year later, my wife got sick for two weeks. I couldn't figure out why. She had recently found a new job and moved into town to join me. She was losing weight, running fevers and feeling horribly fatigued. A visit to her doctor was fruitless. Her physical exam and blood tests were all normal, and the doctor couldn't explain why my wife had had to stop twice to rest on her way up the stairs to his office.

He assured us that she probably had a virus, and that it would pass. With a start, I felt myself mentally transported back a year to that night. I thought about the needlestick—and about what it might mean. If I got sick that was one thing, but my wife? And of course her doctor hadn't tested her for HIV; he'd had no reason to suspect it.

* * * * *

That night, the call room was dark, lit only by a small lamp on the night-stand; the window shades were drawn. I sat on a bed and listened. The din of the hospital had finally faded away. Everything was quiet.

As I looked down at the tourniquet, I knew that what I was about to do might change everything—my job, my health, my sanity.

Such simple objects—a needle, a syringe.

I hesitated for a second. Ethically, I knew I was on shaky ground. I knew that I hadn't thought through all of the possible consequences of tampering with a patient's medical records. I also knew that I couldn't wait until the next day, when I could get a doctor's appointment: I needed to know now.

So I took the plunge.

It was easy to find a label for the vial of blood. In the space where the doctor's signature should go, I scratched an unintelligible scrawl. Then I walked gingerly down the hall to the lab, waited for the desk person to step away for a moment, and left the sample in the drop box.

Back in my call room, I heaved a sigh of relief, cleaned up the wrappers and disposed of the used needle and syringe. My fate, and my wife's, would soon be revealed.

That morning, the attending physician strode toward the nursing station where, with my fellow residents, I waited for him to begin morning rounds.

"Which one of you dumbasses ordered an HIV test on Mr. Jones?" he asked. "Hardly indicated for an eighty-five-year-old man with heart failure."

We all looked at him blankly for a minute. Then I mustered up my courage.

"So when should I start the cocktail of HIV meds?" I asked.

The attending smirked. "*Funny.* It was negative, of course!"

A week later, my wife developed a sore throat. This time, her blood tests showed mono. It would be twelve months before she felt normal again.

* * * * *

Now, ten years having passed, I've thought a lot about what happened and have gained some perspective. Among other things, these events have given me particular empathy for my patients who suffer from chronic illness and the worries and fears they must face on a daily basis.

The training to become a physician is a strange mix of loneliness, fatigue and utter desperation, side by side with the triumphs and achievements of learning to be a healer. The overwhelming stress I felt during my internship altered the way I made decisions.

Now I can see that I was too traumatized by fear and sadness in those early days of residency to find my emotional and professional bearings—and that, as a result, I didn't think clearly or act sensibly. It has taken me years to fully understand that my actions could have had devastating consequences. I could have falsely labeled a patient with HIV. I could have been discovered and dismissed from my residency program.

I realize now that I should have spoken up the minute things started to go wrong—the minute I stuck myself. Most critically, I should have confided in my wife immediately. At the time, I was unable to do this. Looking back, I realize that, for some reason, the process of becoming a doctor created a terrible, unbridgeable divide between me and my non-physician loved ones. I felt that they wouldn't understand my actions and feelings because they hadn't shared my training experiences.

Although I am not proud of my actions—that I didn't confide in my loved ones, that I didn't ask for help—I have forgiven myself. If I were ever faced with such terrifying circumstances again, I hope that the person I have become would think more clearly and act differently this time around, and would realize that I don't need to feel alone.

About the author: *Ken Gordon (a pseudonym) is an aspiring writer, a husband and the father of two beautiful children. He practices "old-fashioned" internal medicine in the suburbs. His poetry has appeared in* Annals of Internal Medicine, Journal of General Internal Medicine *and* The Pharos. *This is his first published story.*

summer

sleep hygiene

Daniel Becker
6/25/2010

Outline the night and all its objects
in black magic marker.

The world through closed eyes
needs texture
the way tires need tread,
brains need wrinkles, and hypnosis
needs the power of suggestion—
traction, surface area, and control
might also apply to a cat
buried alive underneath the sheets;
if so, don't forget the one on top.

Stay up for several nights before
the night you plan to sleep.

Oil the ceiling fan.

True or false: the bladder
is on a separate circuit?

Don't eat in bed, especially chips.

Snoring + sleep apnea + restless legs
+ hemorrhoids + lumbago =

the human condition. The winter itch
as well would be unfair.

Use pillows to solve or suppress all of the above,
a pillow shaped like the horizon
or the supine profile of your partner, or even better
a partner who won't mind being used as a pillow—
together you become the mountains and their clouds,

between the two of you a hidden canyon,
lost in your slopes there are deep limestone caves,
hot springs, the occasional tremor
of tectonic plates and knees.

About the poet: Daniel Becker *practices and teaches general internal medicine and palliative care at the University of Virginia School of Medicine where he also edits the online journal* Hospital Drive. *In August, he teaches at the Taos Writing Retreat for Health Professionals.*

About the poem: "*This poem is an exercise in nonlinear thinking, an attempt to see where 'sleep hygiene' would lead. Around here, most roads lead to or away from the Blue Ridge Mountains.*"

The winner

Majid Khan
7/2/2010

I pull up on the side of the road on this rainy British summer's day. The rain doesn't make it easy to get my doctor's bag out of the trunk, which I do in a hurry so I can make my way to the house where I've been asked to visit a thirty-seven-year-old man named Kenneth.

This really isn't ideal. Now my bag is wet, my papers are wet, my trousers are wet and my mood is wet. I didn't want to do this visit anyway, but I'm still in my last year of training before becoming a full-fledged GP, and I've been given the task by one of the senior GPs in the practice.

"Cough/temperature" says the note the receptionist has scribbled. But while reviewing this patient's records at the surgery I'd also spotted the words "demyelination" and "bed-bound"—words that had triggered my resistance to coming at all.

I knew this visit would upset me. Kenneth has an autoimmune disease like multiple sclerosis that is slowly destroying the sheaths covering his nerves. Kenneth is only nine years older than me.

The brown wooden door opens, and a plump, smiling lady wearing an apron welcomes me in, tells me her name is Charlie and leads me into Kenneth's bedroom, announcing, "The doctor's here."

Kenneth lies in bed on his left side. His muscles, contracted by his disease, allow movement only at a heavy cost in pain. His caregiver, still smiling, returns from the hallway and bustles about him, giving him his medications.

"Easy...Doc...I...might...turn...around...and...smack...ya," says Kenneth, his jovial spirit working its way through paralyzed muscles to reach my very pleasantly surprised ears.

In that moment, I remember my patient Mrs. Beal.

We'd met about two years ago, when I was still a junior doctor. She was a short, white-haired, smiling woman whose zest for life belied her years. Mrs. Beal was always in a good mood—even though she knew we could do nothing to help her. The specialists just didn't know why her kidneys were failing, though they'd asked still other renal specialists for second, third and fourth opinions. All of Mrs. Beal's test results were inconclusive.

I looked forward to seeing her on the ward rounds. She was in the first bed on the left—always smiling, even as she grew increasingly short of breath.

"What's wrong with me, Doc?" she'd occasionally ask querulously. But soon she'd perk up, and we'd be laughing like old friends. As I sat on the end of her bed, she'd ask me about my childhood and why I had become a doctor. So trusting and close was our friendship that she felt comfortable asking, and I felt comfortable answering, questions even about my private dreams and passions. We had discussed things spiritual, mathematics and the enormous power of the mind. And then it was my turn to ask about her life. She adored her children— "*Ohhh,*" she would say, her head turning to the side as if she felt swept away by her devotion.

Powerlessness is perhaps the most powerful feeling a doctor faces. Without any choice in the matter, I'd been thrown into a warm, congenial relationship that I knew had to end. How unfair, I felt, that fate had thrown Mrs. Beal and me together—and how cruel that it would force us to part.

Though she and I never spoke of it, she seemed to know, in those last few days, that her life was heading in only one direction. But that didn't get her down; she always had a smile.

Until the day when I turned up for morning rounds and saw that Mrs. Beal's bed was empty.

They asked me to identify the body. I went to the hospital morgue.

There lay my friend. Death had finally made good on its promise—in spite of all our efforts, in spite of Mrs. Beal's good character, in spite of our friendship and all I'd wanted for her.

As I stood there staring at her snowy hair, amid my grief and anger I felt a silent truth present itself: In the end, you see, *death always wins.*

"You'd...better...fix...me...before...I...go...to the...match..." says Kenneth, pulling me back into the present.

"I'll certainly try, mate," I answer.

Listening to his chest, I hear crackling sounds, and looking through Kenneth's notes I see that this is one of many chest infections for which he's been treated. I find myself wondering whether this will be his last.

I leave a prescription for antibiotics, with instructions to call again if there's no improvement. I shake his stiff hand, bid him farewell and make my way towards the door.

"Are...you...gonna...be...there...Doc?"

"Where?" I say.

"The...match!" he exclaims, incredulous that I have already forgotten what he's likely spent days being excited about.

"Come...on...you...Re...eds!" he says, cheering for his local Birmingham team through smiling, paralyzed lips — in spite of the fact that he can barely move, and that each move costs him heavily in pain; in spite of the fact that he has dreams but may never realize them.

Amid my admiration and sadness, a different, silent truth presents itself: In the end, *life also wins.*

I gather my bag, open the door and head out into the rain.

About the author: *Majid Khan is a general practitioner in Birmingham, UK. He teaches communication skills at Warwick Medical School, where he is also in the process of setting up a course in mindful medical practice and becoming a mindfulness teacher. Another of his stories has appeared in* BJGP: The British Journal of General Practice. *Other personal interests include Buddhism, spirituality and mathematics. He dedicates this story:*

To my books, for teaching me much,
To my teachers, for teaching me much more,
To my patients, for teaching me everything.

trauma in the er

Michael Gutierrez
7/9/2010

It was 5 pm on a cold November day. I was a third-year medical student heading into my first night on surgery call.

Changing into my scrubs, I wondered what it would be like. I knew that we had to carry a "trauma pager" and, when paged, get to the ER as fast as possible. There my job would be to listen as the ER physician called out his exam findings and enter them on a history-and-physical form.

I felt a mix of things. I was excited about the learning possibilities, but I also knew that whoever gets wheeled through the ER doors is someone's daughter, son, mother or father. I decided not to think too hard—I'd just take what came my way and organize my thoughts later.

The night started off slowly. I checked on a patient our team had operated on earlier and added a couple of people to the next day's surgery list. If the evening stayed this mellow, I might have time to study in the call room and get some sleep before rounds the next morning.

Around midnight, my pager went off: "29 y/o female; head on motor vehicle collision; laceration of head; compound fracture of right tibia."

The ER was hushed as the surgery, emergency, orthopedics and nursing teams waited for the patient, some chatting quietly about what the paramedics had told them over the phone. It was like sitting in the eye of a hurricane, knowing that chaos is poised to break through from outside.

Then the patient arrived. She didn't look good: She had an ugly head laceration to go with the fractured tibia, and her systolic blood pressure was in the 40s—too low to sustain life. After minutes that felt like hours, my surgery team took off with her toward the OR for exploratory surgery.

Wheeling her down the hall, I couldn't help remembering that this young woman—a newlywed, I'd just learned—was about my age. We passed her husband and several family members, their eyes filled with heartbreaking fear and sadness.

When we reached the OR, the chief resident called out, "Mike, scrub in, we need you!"

My answering burst of adrenaline reminded me of how I'd felt jumping out of an airplane at 15,000 feet during my first skydive. I was going to learn a lot! But my excitement faded as the enormity of the young woman's situation began to sink in.

Only moments after the first incision, we saw blood spilling out of her liver—so badly ruptured that it was unrecognizable. As the trauma surgeon did his best to stop the hemorrhage, the resident and I pressed our hands to other sites of bleeding. It was difficult to believe that a bit more than an hour ago the purplish clumps running through my fingers had been part of a fully functioning organ.

After an hour of trying, we knew that the woman's injuries were inoperable.

"This isn't working—the bleeding will never stop," my attending told us. "Let's pack in some sponges to slow the bleeding, close her back up and take her to the ICU. I don't want her to die here. I want her to be with her family."

Just ninety minutes ago, I reflected, this woman had been a healthy young newlywed who'd just gotten off the phone with her mother. Then, in one tragic second, her life was over.

Shortly afterwards, I went with my team members to the ICU, where the family members now encircled the patient's bed, looking at her and waiting.

The silence was eerie, broken only by scattered whispers. For me, the loudest noises were my own thoughts as I tried to make sense of what had just happened.

My focus shifted once the attending walked in. It was only a matter of time now before he broke the bad news; then the silence would be pierced by shrieks and sobs.

I found myself wondering how I should act once he'd told the family. Was I supposed to keep my distance and give them space? Or would that seem like indifference? Should I talk to them, express my condolences, even though they looked like they didn't want to be approached? It was confusing.

I decided that, at this stage of my medical career, I should watch my attending to see how he interacted with the family. Witnessing and learning seemed the best I could do.

So, as he spoke quietly with the woman's family, I paid attention from a respectful distance.

"I'm so sorry, we did everything we could," he said gently. "I'm so sorry for your loss."

Tears began to flow, but the family members also seemed appreciative. They gave their permission to take the patient off of life support.

My attending moved to the bedside. Silently, he sat down in a chair, reached over and took the dying young woman's hand. It's an image that will be etched in my mind for the rest of my life.

Sometimes you learn more than you bargained for.

All too often, I realized, we take for granted that we and our loved ones are living, breathing and healthy. All it takes is one instant's misfortune for that to be taken away.

I thought about how I'd sometimes gone weeks on end without communicating with my parents, brother and sister because I had "too much studying to do." I thought about how sad and empty I would feel if a loved one of mine were lying there dying in the ICU, especially if I'd been keeping a distance.

I changed out of my scrubs and headed to my car. Looking back on my weeks of absence as a son, brother and uncle, I asked myself, *Have I become one of those people who's placed his career ahead of his family and loved ones without even realizing it?* The thought was too much to bear.

Pulling up at my apartment complex, I turned off the car engine and reflected.

In that moment, I decided that I was no longer going to make excuses for not being present in the lives of the people closest to me. I realized that my accomplishments mean nothing unless I can share them with those I love.

And I knew that, of the many things I'd learned in my first night of surgery call, this was the biggest lesson of all.

About the author: Michael Gutierrez, originally from Texas, wrote this story in his final year of medical school at the University of Missouri-Kansas City School of Medicine. Michael first became interested in writing as an undergraduate at Pepperdine University. He is an avid reader of historical nonfiction and a dedicated practitioner of Brazilian jujitsu.

Third Party

Mary E. Moore
7/16/2010

Tipping forward to escape
the wheelchair's confines, the ancient one
pleads with her feet, "Go home."

It's her companion who volunteers
the *Chief Complaint*: "Ever since her stroke,
Mother's back seems to hurt.

Her doctors say there's nothing can be done,
but I thought that perhaps a specialist ...."
She strokes the old woman's shoulders.

"Does it hurt here, or there, or if I touch this?"
My fingers probe among birdish bones.
Ignoring me, the patient whimpers, "Home."

When the daughter's eyes register pain, I say,
"I'll inject this spot near her sacroiliac joint.
It may provide relief, in any case do no harm."

I fill in the charge sheet attached to the chart.
Low back pain. Trigger point injection.
*Return PRN.** But how should this be billed?

With the old woman's medical insurance?
With the daughter's?
Or should I pay for this one?

* *PRN is an abbreviation of the Latin phrase* pro re nata, *which in English means "as needed."*

About the poet: *Mary E. Moore earned a PhD as an experimental psychologist, but after working as a research assistant in the psychiatry department of a hospital, she decided to study for an MD. She became a rheumatologist, ultimately heading the Division of Rheumatology at Albert Einstein Medical Center in*

Philadelphia. Since retiring from medicine in 2002, she has been writing poetry. Her poems have been published in many journals and several anthologies and can be seen online at her website, maryemoorepoetry.com.

About the poem: *"This poem reflects a real encounter with a patient. This encounter so impressed me that I wrote about it several years later."*

The cruelest Month

Ray Bingham
7/23/2010

One day in April, I took the assignment none of the other nurses wanted: Baby Michael. A hopeless case.

Born almost four months premature, weighing barely a pound, he was now all of six days old. His entire body wasn't much longer than my open hand. As he lay motionless on a warming bed with the ventilator breathing for him, the night nurse gave me report: serious intestinal infection, bowel surgery, septic shock, multiple antibiotics, infusions to support his failing heart, transfusions to replace the serous drainage seeping from the surgical incision on his darkened, swollen belly.

"Take good care of him," she finished. "He's been through so much already."

As experienced nurses, we both knew that a premature infant rarely survives so many medical complications.

Tiny and sick as he was, his parents Frank and Tonya loved him. Midmorning, they came to visit. They were a young African-American couple—he, tall and wiry; she, shorter, with thick, wavy dark hair. They both looked so weary.

With the attending physician, Dr. Moore, I joined them at Michael's bedside. Trying to be compassionate but honest, we described the progress of Michael's infection and his grave prognosis.

Still, when Tonya held his hand and whispered in his ear, Michael gripped her finger, and his yellowed eyes cracked open.

I remembered a line I'd read in T.S. Eliot's *The Waste Land*—a line borrowed from Shakespeare: "Those are pearls that were his eyes...."

Frank, carrying a small cooler, asked me where the milk freezer was. Together we went to deposit the labeled vials containing Tonya's carefully expressed and frozen drops of yellow-tinged breast milk.

There, in the quiet, Frank said, "I don't know if my wife can take it, seeing our baby this way. But should we stay?" I knew that this was his way of asking me how soon his son would die.

"While Michael's alive, there's always hope," I replied. "But he's small and weak. He's been through a lot."

We returned to Michael's bedside.

Frank and Tonya sat together, holding each other and whispering softly to their son. After a short while, they said their goodbyes and left.

For the rest of the day, Michael made no response as I turned him, stroked his cheek or suctioned his breathing tube. I changed his diaper only out of a sense of ritual. It was dry; his bowels and kidneys had shut down.

Seven o'clock came. The night-shift nurses entered the unit.

At least I won't be the one taking Michael to the morgue, I thought.

At that moment, his heart rate began to drift down. The monitor alarm rang. My fellow nurses rushed over with the emergency cart containing meds, tubes, needles and the defibrillator with its tiny neonatal electrode pads.

Another line from Eliot's poem came to me: "I have heard the key turn in the door once and turn once only."

It was time to turn the key and let Michael go.

"Don't touch him," I said.

Just then, Dr. Moore appeared. "What's going on?"

"We talked about this on rounds this morning," I answered. "We're already doing everything we can. At this point, we're just causing him more pain."

"Ray, I sympathize, but we have no choice," said Dr. Moore. "We have to do this." Although Frank and Tonya had discussed the DNR (do not resuscitate) order, they hadn't been able to bring themselves to sign it.

I looked at Michael. I had the sense that he'd departed long since—perhaps when his parents had left. He was already beyond our reach.

Reluctantly, I nodded and took my place by his side. The code proceeded—chest compressions, bag ventilation, messy blood draws for STAT lab work, hurried intravenous lines for more access, shocks from the defibrillator jolting his tiny torso.

Then at last it was over.

I looked down at the bloodied bedsheet, the red-spattered equipment, the tiny, bruised body.

Again Eliot's words came to me: "April is the cruelest month..."

I wiped up the spilled blood, changed the spattered linens and took away the equipment.

Responding to our phone call, Frank and Tonya rushed in as I was bathing Michael's swollen body. Dr. Moore took them to the conference room.

I finished the bath, dressed and wrapped the body, made the bed with clean linens and pulled the screens around it. At last, I went to join Michael's parents.

I found them seated in the dim room, Dr. Moore leaning forward, Tonya sobbing on the couch as Frank held her.

"I'd like to see him," Frank told me.

I walked him to the bed. Frank looked at his son, clean and swaddled, a blue knitted cap on his head, and asked me to take a last picture of Michael lying there peacefully, as if sleeping.

"I don't think Tonya should see him," Frank said. "It might hurt her too much."

"Your wife is strong," I answered. "She'll need to work through her own grief."

So I lifted Michael from the bed and carried him to the back. Tonya took him from me and held him, crying. Then she smiled, recounting the details of their son's brief struggle with life. She thanked us.

"He felt your love," I said. "The last thing I saw him do was to grip your finger and open his eyes."

And again, I remembered the pearls that were his eyes.

About the author: Ray Bingham lives in Gaithersburg, MD, with his wife, three kids, three cats and one dog. He worked as a neonatal nurse for more than ten years before turning his attention to science writing and editing. His essays and stories have appeared in a wide range of publications, including The Washington Post, Health Affairs, American Journal of Nursing *and* Journal of Nursing Jocularity. *He is an avid, if not particularly fast, runner.*

james and bob

Paul Rousseau
7/30/2010

I think his name was James, but I can't remember for sure. What I do remember is the day's heat, the metal cart and a rust-colored dog.

Like many homeless people, James carried his belongings in a grocery cart—a sort of mobile home for the homeless, but without the protection of a roof, the support of four walls or the security of a front door.

I'd just walked out of the local Safeway store into its parking lot. He ambled over from a park across the street. His eyes were narrow, his face tanned and his clothes dirty brown from weeks of sleeping in the streets.

Being a dog lover, I found my eyes drawn to the dog—a mixed breed with matted hair, worn eyes and gray hairs on his snout. He looked underweight; I guessed he weighed no more than thirty or forty pounds. He stood obediently by James' side, tethered by a rope leash.

"What's his name?" I asked.

"He's Bob—best dog there is. In fact, best friend a man could have," said James in a deep smoker's voice. He smiled and rubbed Bob's back.

Then he asked, "Can you give me some money so I can get some food?"

How many times had I been asked this question in this exact same Safeway parking lot? And how many times had I answered "No!" and kept walking?

But this time felt different. James looked emaciated, and his plea seemed honest.

"Is the food for you, Bob, or both of you?" I asked.

"For both of us," he answered.

I thought for a moment, and then told James to tell me what he needed; I would go inside and get it for him. That way, I thought, he couldn't buy alcohol, cigarettes or drugs, and I would be sure that he and Bob would have a decent meal, at least for today.

James agreed and spouted off a small list.

After buying the groceries, I went back outside; James and Bob had seemingly disappeared. Looking around, I spotted them back in the park, walked over and sat down beside them. I handed James the groceries and filled two bowls for Bob—one with food, one with water.

As they both ate, I somehow felt comfortable enough with James to ask how he'd ended up homeless and wandering the streets of Phoenix with Bob at his side.

He told me he'd been a long-distance truck driver, with the truck being his only home for the past twenty or so years. For even longer, he'd also been a four- to five-pack-a-day smoker, and an admitted lover of anything alcoholic.

"But I never drove when I was drunk," he said firmly. My brows raised in disbelief.

About six months back, while driving through Texas on a haul from Florida to California, he'd noticed he was shorter of breath than usual. When he coughed, bloody phlegm streaked his handkerchief of toilet paper. He'd continued driving through Amarillo and Albuquerque, then down I-17 to Phoenix. By the time he'd arrived in Phoenix, there were blood clots in the tissue, so he'd parked his rig at one of the local hospitals, checked into the emergency room and waited his turn.

Initially they'd been worried about a blood clot in his lung, given the long periods he spent sitting behind the wheel of his rig, so they ordered a CT scan.

"What did they find?" I asked.

"The doctor told me there were spots all over my lung. When I asked what that meant, he told me they looked like cancer."

Another CT scan done at the same time showed suspicious lesions in James' liver and "glands." The doctor referred James to an oncologist, but he had no insurance, wasn't from Phoenix and felt scared. It was then that he walked away from the rig, leaving it in the hospital parking lot, and began his homeless journey throughout the city of Phoenix and the surrounding suburbs.

"I wanted to live my final days free, not bothering anyone, not a burden to anyone."

I asked about his family. He'd been married once and had no children. Where his wife was now he had no idea. His parents were dead. He had two sisters, but didn't know their whereabouts.

I asked where he got Bob.

"One day I was walking through Glendale and found this scraggy mutt wandering the streets," James said. That was six months ago, and they'd been inseparable since.

He had only one concern about his illness: "I worry so much about what will happen to Bob."

Tears welled up in his eyes. He'd probably have to take him to a shelter, he said; he didn't trust anyone on the streets to care for Bob after he was gone.

I asked if I could help in any way—maybe try to get him in to see a physician—but he declined. I asked about hospice, wondering if any of the local hospices would take in a nomadic man with no address. Many times hospices will provide free care, I explained, and I would gladly see what I could do for him, because while he was able to get around now, his ability to care for himself would surely diminish in the future.

Again James declined, but thanked me for my concern. Then he stood, thanked me for the groceries and said it was time for he and Bob to hit the road and find a place for the night.

"I appreciate your help, I surely do. God bless you."

He tugged at Bob and headed down an embankment toward the nearby highway bridge.

They both turned, gave me one last look and disappeared underneath.

I wondered if the story I'd just heard was true. But James had looked sick, and his story seemed legitimate; my heart begged me to believe it. What did he have to gain by telling such a story? Why would he lie?

I walked across the street and sat in my car for a few minutes, the cool, air-conditioned breeze blowing in my face. I vowed then to change things—to become an advocate for the homeless and terminally ill. I even envisioned finding some philanthropist to donate money so that I could provide hospice services at the homeless shelter.

But, like many dreams, this one dried up under the heat of the Phoenix sun and the demands of my own personal life. There were the long hours at work, the demands of caring for my daughters after the death of their mother, and the burden of my own grief.

I never saw James and Bob again, although I often looked for them. But to this day, their presence remains in my mind, a picture of loneliness, stubborn pride, bravery and the love between a man and a dog.

And maybe, just maybe, one day I'll develop that hospice for the homeless—and their dogs—with the things many of them so desperately need: the protection of a roof, the support of four walls and the security of a front door.

About the author: *Paul Rousseau is associate professor of internal medicine and geriatrics at the Medical University of South Carolina, and medical director of its palliative and supportive care program. A hospice and palliative-care physician for the past thirty years, he has had some 350 pieces published in* Annals of Internal Medicine, JAMA, Blood and Thunder *and elsewhere. "I've been* *writing my whole life, but I have used writing as therapy ever since the death of my wife. I enjoy writing about the patients and families who allow me the honor of entering their lives at such a frightening and vulnerable time."*

Dissolution

Jocelyn Jiao
8/6/2010

the articles went first.
then the pronouns, the verbs,
nouns. they melted away, leaving
only memories of warmth
cradled by salivary glands.
adjectives flutter behind
my front teeth, ready for flight.
only adverbs remain,
curled beneath my tongue—
yawning, drowsy:
the softest words of vocabulary.

the lilt of my voice has left too,
soapy Californian vowels
scrubbed clean.
when i speak to my mother,
she complains of my consonants,
how they have begun
to iron out cadences, climb
over inflections, ride
them into deep sand. she says
only my whisper remains whole.
but not for long;
already the throat whistles.

it all started at your
bedside, when your lips
were parted, straining
to form one first, final word.
a sudden embrace of cold
concrete made you into
some bright thing with eyes
translucent, gasping
for the comfort of
water, empty and clear—

when ebullience
once spilled from your lips
as a sun warms an earth.

do you see? words are meant
for creatures of air. i have no use for them;
even fish can sing.

gently, carefully, tenderly,
night arrives; it pivots and
provides no answer. i feel your name
coil in my mouth, watch
as it ebbs away
with the receding waters.

About the poet: Jocelyn Jiao wrote this poem as an undergraduate at Stanford University. She has since graduated with a bachelor of arts degree in human biology.

About the poem: "Language is probably the most precious of gifts. Without it, we are utterly alone—smothered and helpless. While not all of us may have experienced the same kind of loss, we all have lost something. I think we can all relate to how, at the most terrible and profound of times, what comes immediately is not a shout or scream. Words escape us. Bodies take charge; they force us to mourn, properly, in silence."

Angels and phantoms

Joanna Dognin
8/13/2010

"Mama," a little voice pipes from the back seat. "Why is that boy in a chair?"

The sun is beaming into the car as we sit at a stoplight, waiting to exit a store parking lot. My two-year-old daughter has spotted a young man, barely twenty, who smiles weakly as he rolls by in an electric wheelchair, collecting money for muscular dystrophy.

"He's in a chair because he needs help moving around," I say.

"Why?"

"Because his legs need help."

"Why? Because they don't work?"

"Well..."

"Why are they broken?" she asks. "Is he broken? Why is he here? Where is his mama? Mama, where is the boy's mama?"

* * * * *

"Dr. Lobozzo, you got any kids?" Gabriel asked, calling me by my maiden name rather than the married name I'd only recently begun using.

"No," he continued with a sly smile. "Don't tell me. I already know. You have two sons."

I was newly married (without children), living in one of New York City's boroughs and working in the city's outer boroughs and working in a primary-care center I'd joined after getting my psychology license. The center integrated mental health and social services into primary care.

I had been seeing Gabriel for three years. Once a week he'd come for psychotherapy, braving a two-bus commute in a clunky, red electric wheelchair, adorned with a horn that he'd toot to announce his arrival. The chair also sported a flag, bumper stickers and assorted other trinkets given to him by his home health aide, a heavy-set woman he affectionately called "Mama Rosa."

Twenty-two years earlier, Gabriel had been born HIV-positive. His mother had been neglectful, if not abusive, so he'd spent his childhood shuttling from one foster home to another. Gabriel's chronically poor health had gone unnoticed and untreated until his adolescence, when a sudden stroke led to a prolonged hospitalization, discovery of his HIV status and a strained reconnection with his mother—now also known to be HIV-positive—and older siblings.

When I first met Gabriel, he was already very ill. His T-cell-less body had withstood cryptosporidium, toxoplasmosis and just about every other opportunistic infection. He lived in a nursing home, cared for by an assortment of home health aides. His family contacts were limited to occasional phone calls and (broken) promises of visits. The resulting isolation caused him constant distress and longing.

Understandably, Gabriel's caregivers had become his surrogate family. As he grew sicker and weaker, he turned more and more to his doctor and to me for nurturance, fantasizing about the rich family lives we supposedly led.

Therapy was challenging: Gabriel vacillated between a wish for life, for family, for meaning, and an inner pull towards despair and death. In some therapy sessions he talked about the future, especially one where he might someday have a wife and children. In many others he spoke incessantly of his impending death.

Sadly, maddeningly, as his mood swung up or down, so did his adherence to his HIV medication regimen. When feeling more hopeful, he'd take the life-saving drugs; in darker times, he'd stop. He was often hospitalized for what was expected to be the last time, but somehow he'd always bounce back.

Gabriel's doctor and I did our best, through counseling, to help Gabriel break this self-destructive cycle. When our efforts failed, we became more like insistent parents pleading with an unwilling child.

Through it all, Gabriel's health grew steadily worse—and his fantasies of my "sons" more vivid. During this last hospital stay, he imagined me leaving his bedside to run home and care for them.

"I know you have to go, right? Or maybe you can stay?" he asked weakly, then continued, "I bet your sons are waiting for you at home to cook for them. I bet they want their pasta, Dr. Lobozzo."

"Yes, I need to go soon," I responded quietly, glancing at a nurse in the corridor and then looking out the window. The hot July sun was fading slowly into early evening. I saw Central Park in the distance and thought longingly of going for a solitary evening run. I looked back at Gabriel, wishing that his mother were here to reprieve me of the heaviness in the room and wondering how much the very pressure of his need kept her at bay.

Trying to bridge the distance between Gabriel and his absent mother, I'd often left messages inviting her to a family session, and the hospital staff had called her each time he was admitted. Yet she never showed. In fact, I'd never even spoken directly with her on the phone. Wrestling with Gabriel's bottomless, unmet needs, I struggled to find some empathy for this shadowy woman who'd caused her child so much pain.

He'd been looking forward to this summer, to spending his favorite August days sitting outside, watching the world go by—but he was also growing sicker and sicker. The previous Christmas, he'd brought us gifts: a blanket for his doctor, whose hands were always cold; a bottle of olive oil for me, "to cook a nice Italian meal for your boys." In his own way, I think, he knew he had no more Christmases left.

"It's okay, you can go," Gabriel sighed. "It's late, and your sons must be hungry." Maybe he needed an excuse for why I didn't stay longer, as a devoted mother might. Or maybe he imagined himself sitting next to his brothers at our dinner table, eating the meal he'd helped to prepare.

Gently, I said goodbye and left.

After my visit, we again called Gabriel's mother, who again did not show up. She was, I reflected, becoming as much of a phantom to me as my "sons."

I went on vacation at the end of that long, hot summer, while Gabriel was still in the hospital. And while I was away, he died. I can still taste my disbelief: the shock that this ending, so long anticipated, had happened so briskly during my few days away.

The hospital staff told me that, in Gabriel's last days, his mother appeared. I still wonder what words and gestures passed between them at the end. I hope that he felt nurtured and mothered in the ways he most needed, and by the person whose caring he most craved. Above all, I hope their time together brought them both peace.

I would have liked to meet Gabriel's mother—to have had a chance to understand her absence before Gabriel faded away and I too moved on. But perhaps this was selfish. Maybe it was better that Gabriel's final moments with his mother, brief as they were, be private.

* * * * *

The traffic light turns to green. We leave the young man in the wheelchair.

"Mama," chimes my daughter.

My thoughts of Gabriel fade. Driving up the hill, I brace myself for more questions.

"Mama," she repeats. "The boy is gone....But look!" she shouts brightly. "I can see the moon! Mama, does the moon wear pajamas?"

I look back at my smiling child and her sleeping baby brother, and my heart breaks just a little bit. I'm struck by how easily what we love can be lost. Our ghosts and our living loved ones dance together across time and place, teaching us to be stronger parents, therapists and people.

Now Gabriel is a phantom—a boy sitting in a wheelchair and smiling a big, goofy smile, a boy who just wanted his mother—and the two children he imagined are real. They toddle through the world, happy and strong, and blissfully unaware of angels and phantoms, of mothers leaving children and of babies born broken and reaching out for mothers all around them.

About the author: Joanna Dognin is a clinical psychologist who has worked in primary-care settings for the past ten years. She currently works at the Veterans Administration NY Harbor on health promotion and disease prevention initiatives. She is a clinical assistant professor in the department of psychiatry of New York University School of Medicine.

Dr. B gets an F

Gregory Shumer
8/20/2010

Flashback to a year ago: I'm a first-year medical student—a fledgling, a novice—trying to integrate countless facts into a coherent understanding of how the human body works. Professors slam me with two months' worth of information inside of two weeks' time. They tell us that this is a necessary process, one that all doctors must go through: We must first learn the science of medicine before we can master the art of healing.

My life revolves around tests, labs, deadlines, long hours in the library and very close relationships with the baristas at Starbucks.

In the midst of this chaos, I developed a crippling ankle condition that transformed me into a concerned patient for the first time in my life. The pain started as a dull ache that I experienced only during exercise. Then it gradually worsened, to the point where I could barely walk to school the day after I'd played a basketball game. A golf-ball-sized bulge stuck out from my right ankle, and my two months of medical education suggested no remedies.

It was at this point—worried, looking for answers and desperate to get back to normal—that I decided to see someone.

Dr. B, the orthopedist I consulted, had attended a prestigious medical school and had gone on to complete an illustrious residency program and a fellowship specializing in the foot and ankle. I waited thirty minutes in the exam room before he walked in, flanked by a second-year resident wearing a long white coat. Dr. B himself wore a gray sports jacket and tie. His hair was slicked back, and he radiated authority.

After introducing himself, he glanced at my x-rays and MRI and started examining my ankles.

"You see this," he said to his resident. "I can fit my two fingers underneath his left foot, but none under his right. This patient has been running his arch into the ground." Glancing back at me, he told me to walk in a straight line.

As I walked, he said to the resident, "Yup, look at that. He's pronating way too much on his right side. Something's off with the mechanics there."

He went on talking to the resident, never addressing his comments to me, and using medical terms that I didn't understand.

Finally, scribbling in my chart, he said, "Sit down."

I sat, feeling confused.

"All right," he said, "I'm going to order you some rehab, and I want you to get a pair of orthotics. Rest your ankle, and come back and see me in five months."

He handed me the chart, stood up and turned to leave.

"When you say 'rest my ankle,' what does that mean exactly?" I asked his back. "I was hoping to play basketball in a few weeks, and I want to run a 5K a couple of months from now."

Turning back and grinning wryly, he said, "I wouldn't do any running until you see me again. The way your ankle looks, I'm more concerned with your walking normally at age thirty-five than running in a 5K next month. Any other questions?"

He seemed annoyed at being delayed. For my part, I felt panicky. What had seemed like a small problem now seemed like much, much more.

"Is surgery an option?" I asked.

He paused, then said it was risky and probably not the best idea.

My mind was racing. I couldn't bear the thought of giving up physical activity—one of the few pleasures in my life of stress and studying. But I asked no more questions, for fear of irritating him further.

Dr. B turned again, opened the door and walked out.

My visit to Dr. B was the worst encounter I'd ever had with a physician. I'd gone in seeking answers, guidance and direction. I came out feeling scared, confused and worried that I would never be the same on my feet again.

I didn't make a follow-up appointment .

I did start physical therapy, as he'd recommended, and I made an appointment with a podiatrist recommended by a friend.

The physical therapist was wonderful. And he was incredulous when I told him of Dr. B's concerns about my ability to walk later in life.

"A doctor told you that?" he said. "I've seen people with worse problems than yours recover 100 percent. And you're young! With rehab and stretching, we can have you running and playing basketball again. I'm confident of that."

I left the session with a plan for my recovery, and feeling a lot more hopeful.

Then I saw the podiatrist, Dr. Stevenson. Podiatrists attend podiatry school instead of medical school and are trained in the diagnosis and treatment of foot and ankle conditions. When I repeated Dr. B's words to him, he looked at me and said, "You know, I've seen hundreds of people with problems worse than yours, and you know how many I've told they would never run again?"

I shrugged.

"Zero," he said, making a circle with his thumb and forefinger.

After having me walk in several straight lines, he studied my feet and ankles for a long time. He showed me an anatomical model and explained what was going on: My arch had started to collapse and apply extra pressure on an already injured posterior tibialis tendon. With rest and the help of an orthotic device, the tendon could heal—and I could return to running and playing sports. He then sat down and answered all of my questions; I had plenty. I left feeling much more optimistic about my condition.

Being a patient and seeing three different professionals gave me valuable insights into the doctor-patient relationship. Although Dr. B had attended prestigious schools and on paper had more qualifications than the physical therapist or podiatrist, his lack of compassion and poor communication skills made him a far inferior clinician.

I promised myself at that point, while still a beginning medical student, that I'd never practice medicine like Dr. B. I want to be a caring physician who not only makes the correct diagnosis but also facilitates the healing process by listening to, reassuring and working with patients.

In my first year of medical school, when the focus had been on memorizing medical and anatomical facts, my own anatomy managed to teach me a pointed clinical lesson without any cramming at all.

A year later, many of the facts I stuffed into my head are lost to me, but that lesson has stayed. It had better—if I'm to be the kind of doctor that I myself would want to go to.

About the author: *Gregory Shumer is a medical student at Georgetown University School of Medicine, class of 2013. After graduating from the University of Michigan with a degree in Biology and Asian Studies in 2008, Gregory spent a year teaching English to middle-school students in rural Japan. He started writing essays, poems and short stories in high school and now continues to enjoy writing as a medical student. He looks forward to his future career as a family physician.*

chirality

Stacy Nigliazzo
8/27/2010

I see myself, always
through a stark looking glass

the fun house view of my own face
reflected in the eyes of my patients—

> tangled in the bleeding strands
> that line the gray sclera of the meth addict

> drowning in the pooling ink that splits
> the swelling pupil of the hemorrhagic stroke

> swimming in the antibiotic slather
> that blurs the newborn's first gaze—

my clouded countenance,
ever present—

> slipping even through parched flesh
> along the steely glide of the angiocath

> glistening in the fluid bag
> of intravenous medication

> glaring back
> from the sliding metal siderail—

twelve hours streaming from my skin
like an open wound in the scrub sink

face to face
in the soap-splattered mirror—

only then,
do I look away.

About the poet: *Stacy Nigliazzo is a poet and ER nurse. Her work has been featured in* JAMA, *the* American Journal of Nursing, Third Space *and the* Bellevue Literary Review, *among other publications. A graduate of Texas A&M University, she is a recipient of the Elsevier Award for Nursing Excellence. Her poem "Relic" was a finalist for the 2012 Marica and Jan Vilcek poetry prize.*

About the word: " *'Chirality' refers to the quality of some objects that cannot be superimposed upon their mirror images. According to* Wikipedia, *'Human hands are perhaps the most universally recognized example of chirality: The left hand is a non-superposable mirror image of the right hand; no matter how the two hands are oriented, it is impossible for all the major features of both hands to coincide. This difference in symmetry becomes obvious if…a left-handed glove is placed on a right hand.'* "

About the poem: *"In an emergency setting, the interventions provided by nurses are often harsh by nature (inserting large-bore IV lines, etc.). Other times, there is nothing that can be done except to provide comfort as a patient deteriorates. This poem is a personal exploration of the difficulty and responsibility of this role, as well as an attempt to catch a glimpse of my patients' perceptions of me as a nurse and my own perceptions of myself."*

Broken

Jordan Grumet
9/3/2010

I was a third-year medical student in the first week of my obstetrics rotation. The obstetrics program was known to be high-pressure, its residents among the best. Mostly women, they were a hard-core group—smart, efficient, motivated—and they scared the heck out of us medical students.

I remember the day clearly: Not only was I on call, but I was assigned to the chief resident's team. I felt petrified.

We'd started morning rounds as usual, running down the list of patients in labor. Five minutes in, my chief got a "911" page from the ER, located in the next building. This seldom happened, so instead of calling back, we ran downstairs and over to the trauma bay.

We walked into pure chaos. The patient was twenty-seven, in her last weeks of pregnancy and actively exsanguinating—bleeding to death. She and her husband had been fighting; apparently he'd picked up a kitchen knife and stabbed her in the neck.

As the ER physician and the trauma surgeon worked rapidly on the woman's neck, my chief readied herself to deliver the baby. She turned to me.

"Quick, get me a sterile gown and a scalpel."

Helping her to gown and glove, I could see the other physicians getting coated by the blood spurting from the women's neck. She'd been talking when she arrived by ambulance; she wasn't talking anymore.

The nurses were pumping blood into large-bore IVs in both of her arms, but the patient's blood pressure kept dropping. On the fetal monitor, we saw the baby's heart rate starting to dip.

My chief cleared her throat: "Okay, guys, we're gonna lose the baby if we don't do something fast!"

Without taking his eyes from the patient, the trauma surgeon said authoritatively, "We can't. If you cut her, she'll die. Give us a minute."

"It will take a minute-and-a-half to have this baby out," said my chief. She got no answer.

She stood poised over the patient's abdomen, arm raised, scalpel in hand and ready to pounce.

The patient's blood pressure dropped even faster, and the baby's heart rate plummeted.

"It's now or never," said my chief. Then the cardiac monitor began beeping.

"Ventricular fibrillation!" The ER physician grabbed the cardiac paddles and shouted, "Clear!"

With a sweep of his arm, the trauma surgeon moved everyone away from the table, then stepped back—and crashed into my chief. She fell to the floor, extending her arm to avoid slashing anyone with the scalpel.

The electrical shocks, delivered over the course of several minutes, didn't revive the patient. Her wavy cardiac tracing flattened into one long, straight line.

By then it was too late to save the baby. Its heart rate had been too low for too long, causing severe, irreversible brain damage. As we listened, the fetal monitor went silent.

The walk back to the obstetrics floor was eerily quiet. I wanted somehow to comfort the chief...to comfort myself...but I didn't know how. As we reached the nursing station, she slowly came unwound.

For the first hour, all she wanted to do was talk. She grabbed every resident and nurse who walked by, going over and over what had happened. If only she had disregarded the trauma surgeon, things could have been different....

Then she became intensely quiet. She sat at the table in the middle of the nursing station, her face contorting into a myriad of expressions as she mentally replayed the events. Occasionally she raised her right arm as if wielding the scalpel again.

Finally, she put her head down and started to cry—loud, disconcerting sobs. The staff and patients passed to and fro, largely ignoring her. No one seemed to know how to comfort such a strong, accomplished physician in her time of need.

And there I stood—helpless in a sea of sadness and pain.

She cried for what seemed liked hours. Then she picked up the phone, made a call, placed her pager on the table and left the hospital.

A few minutes later, an attending came in to replace her, to pick up the pager and to collect me.

The next day, my chief returned to work. She acted as if nothing had happened. No mention was made of the day before.

She finished the year and is now a well-known attending physician at a prestigious medical center.

I'll always remember that day as the day that medicine broke her—destroyed her innocence. To me, she seemed like a soldier who had witnessed her first death in battle. Would she ever be the same? Or had she lost a sacred part of herself forever?

I feel sure that this is what happened because I remember when medicine broke me—one lonely night, watching helplessly as a patient died in the intensive care unit. I'd bet that most of my colleagues have had similar experiences. We rarely talk about them, but you might get some answers if you asked our loved ones.

They would tell you how we changed over the course of our medical training. How one day we came home from work seeming different. How a young, eager, empathic man or woman gradually became angry, frustrated and often cold. How we started out suffering *with* our patients, but ended up suffering *from* them.

And that's the paradox of medicine. We enter this profession out of a passion to help others. But repeated exposure to the most agonizing situations causes pain that can make us retreat into a shell of cynicism or "clinical objectivity." There, we risk losing the softness, warmth and caring that sent us into medicine in the first place.

Now, years later, I know that some of us—the lucky ones—recover. For me, the anger and frustration started to reverse six years ago with the birth of my son. Gradually, I learned to tend the wounds that medicine had inflicted on me. Now I'm no longer so scared of being hurt. Now I can cry with my patients, not because of them.

And now I finally feel like the physician I'd always hoped to be—a little more caring, a little more loving and a little less afraid of what the future will bring.

About the author: Jordan Grumet is an assistant professor at the University of Chicago and practices internal medicine in the Chicago suburbs. He writes as an outlet—in response to his often busy and sometimes stressful medical practice.

Falling in Love with My Doctor

Judith Lieberman
9/10/2010

The other doctors I consulted called him brilliant. His past patients praised his compassion. He actually responded to e-mails. And, lastly, he was known as the best-looking doctor at the cancer center. What more could I ask?

On the other hand, what choice did I have? After twelve years, I was facing a recurrence of a relatively rare oral cancer, located inconveniently at the base of my tongue. The treatment options were not great. The radical surgery recommended by one prominent cancer center could have left me unable to swallow, talk or eat normally.

My incredible husband stayed up many nights researching surgery, radiation, chemotherapy and all the combinations. On the bright side, my teenagers cleaned their rooms without being asked!

The last straw came when, while talking on my cell phone to yet another cancer center and making the turn into a parking lot, I crashed my car. Just one more broken item needing to be fixed.

* * * * *

I prepare for eight weeks of combined chemotherapy and radiation, which my new doctor candidly describes as "setting off a bomb in your mouth." Sitting in the exam room, I know that my husband is paying close attention as the doctor shows us the details of my uncooperative oral anatomy on his computer screen.

But I am watching my doctor.

His eyes are brown, and they look directly into mine while he speaks. His voice is calm, and his hands are firm and warm when they touch me. My heart flutters, and I feel like a schoolgirl, excited and shy.

It certainly feels much better to have a crush than to have cancer.

I decide to go along for the ride. I buy "lounge wear" to replace office casual, and a fancy overnight bag for hospital trips. My husband buys me a

Kindle so I can download books from my anticipated sickbed. We stock the kitchen with Jell-O and flaxseed oil, easy to swallow and full of purported healing powers.

* * * * *

Several weeks and many radiation treatments later, I am back at the cancer center for another all-day chemotherapy session. I am attached to the IV, have only half my hair and "eat" nutritional glop via a stomach tube. (My teenage daughter rationalizes this as the ultimate in body piercing.) My neck is raw, and I do my best to cover it with a variety of cheery scarves. I have that delightful "chemo grey" complexion.

One late afternoon, I wake from restless sleep to see my doctor sitting in the corner. The curtains are drawn, and he is writing on a chart in the room's only shaft of light, waiting patiently to talk to me. He looks up. His sad eyes meet mine, and he smiles at me.

At that moment I fall in love.

I fall in love with hope. It pulls me through the weeks of being unable to eat, days where my only goal is to make it to the next day, and moments of pain that must be endured. I remember this instant clearly as my entry into a place beyond my rational experience.

* * * * *

Eventually, though, after weeks and months in this nameless place, the intensity of my feelings shifts. I begin to eat again, and I wean myself from the narcotics and medications. I throw away the scarves and the "sick clothes." My prognosis improves, and I return joyously to the routines of daily life, with my ability to eat and speak intact.

I begin to arrive at my doctor appointments late instead of early, and my beloved doctor now has new patients whose situations are more dire and urgent than mine.

For cancer patients, and many others, the doctor-patient relationship is as delicate and complex as that of any pair of lovers. You, my physician, know the secrets of my body in the most strangely intimate ways. I submit willingly. It was important for me to fall in love, to cling intensely to you as I traveled this strange road—to trust totally in our relationship and believe with all my heart.

I don't know if my doctor knew about the wild love affair I had with him. For me, the boundaries changed as I struggled with death, disease and suffering. Ultimately, I know that my doctor loves his work in a profound way. In so doing, he made me feel loved.

I hope it was okay that I loved him back.

About the author: Judy Lieberman lives in the San Francisco Bay Area and has written all her life for work, pleasure and the amusement of her friends and family. Anyone interested in the oral cancer journey can visit her blog at http://jlwordofmouth.blogspot.com. *"It seems that many medical professionals beat themselves up a lot. A part of what I wanted to convey in this piece is that we (patients with serious illness) know that doctors and nurses are also only human."*

Life, preciously poured

Kate Benham
9/17/2010

You pour a cup of pecans
Like a kid catching raindrops
In a bucket.
Careful not to spill,
Your fingers playing tremolo on a
Violin-string cup measure.

Your bed-tucked
Mouth, warm, with
Tongue searching the lips
For forgotten first lines of bedtime stories
Like misplaced glasses, resting on your head.
I read to you, now,
In hospital beds.

Forehead wrinkles stacked
In three creases—
Your crossword face,
Mouth-chewed pencil between your lips,
Scooping for synonyms
As you now scoop sugar.

Patient tablespoons of vanilla
Heaped with the effort
Of standing up for fifteen minutes

Love spelled in spilled flour
By hairless eyelid blinks.

This mother's day coffee cake
Streuseled with memories of able-bodied bike rides
Suspended in white hospital gauze.
It tastes like antiseptic and cinnamon.
This baking is labor
For the hands of a heart surgeon
Too tremored to hold a scalpel,

Hold a measuring cup,
Hold on.

His life
Preciously poured,
Savored in my mouth
Even as it slides down
My throat—
Swallowed.

About the poet: Kate Benham *wrote this as an undergraduate at Stanford University; she graduated in 2009 with a BA in feminist studies. Afterwards, she worked for* The Clayman Institute for Gender Research *on a project about social bias in medical and basic science research, and lived in India for one year. She is currently a second-year medical student at Columbia University College of Physicians and Surgeons.*

About the poem: "During my senior year of college, my father was diagnosed with multiple myeloma, a type of bone-marrow cancer. I started writing as a way of processing the feelings I felt I couldn't share with any of my peers, as so few were experiencing similar circumstances."

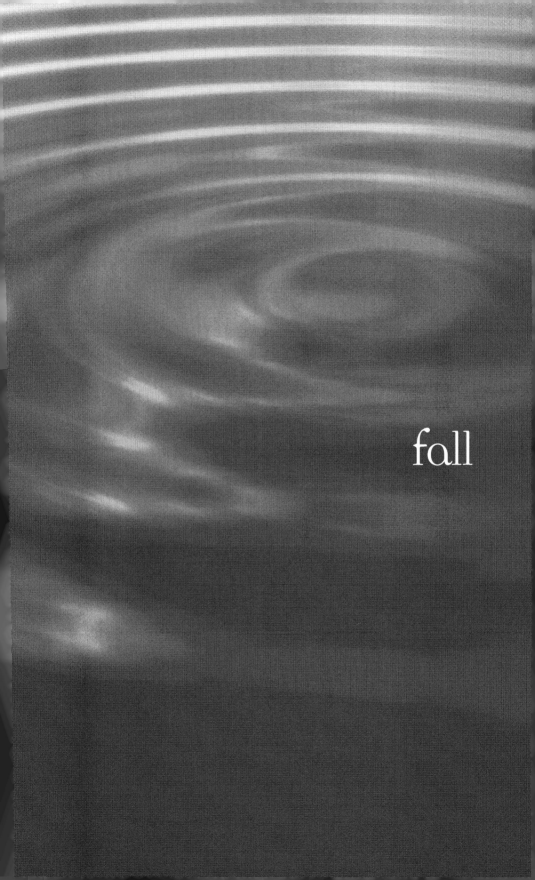

fall

affected

Jessica Tekla Les
9/24/2010

During my third year of medical school I was performing a routine breast exam, more for practice than anything else. I was trying the concentric-circles-around-the-nipple technique, one of several I'd been taught. About halfway through the right breast I found a lima-bean-sized lump, not far from the breastbone. I took liberties with this particular exam. I poked the lump, tried to move the lump, squished down on the lump.

I took such liberties because it was my own breast.

At the time, I responded clinically. I thought to myself, *I am twenty-seven years old, with no family history and no risk factors. Nothing to worry about.* I knew the likely diagnosis, a fibroadenoma or localized fibrocystic change, both common in my age group. I double-checked a textbook to be sure, then dismissed the lump from my mind.

A month later, shortly after my twenty-eighth birthday, my primary-care doctor stumbled upon the lump during an annual physical—even though I hadn't mentioned it to her. She agreed that the lump was tender and freely mobile, the opposite of what a cancer should feel like, but she ordered an ultrasound, just to be safe.

I thought, *Really?*

Then fear crept in.

Five long weeks later, my biopsy results confirmed breast cancer, catapulting me from doctor-in-training to patient in one nauseating instant. My breast surgeon delivered the news with honesty and tenderness, but I felt desperate to escape that house of bad news and go somewhere else, even if only to another clinical building for the MRI that she'd ordered to determine the cancer's size.

I crossed the pavement and ducked out of the late summer twilight and into the imaging building's fluorescently lit halls. But in this new building I found no relief. The receptionist stamped my name and medical-record number on a stack of consent forms, then handed them to me. Turning to find a seat, I ran smack up against the absurd side of my diagnosis: the garish waiting-room artwork on the walls.

As I waited for my name to be called, my sister and friends came to join me. Together we deliberated, then voted, on which painting was most hideous. There was no question: the abstract horses dancing amid lurid pastel brushstrokes.

Since it was a Friday night, the MRI technician had some trouble cajoling a radiology resident into coming downstairs to put an IV into me. Walking down the hall, the resident swaggered in his scrubs like an underwear model. But once holding the needle, he quivered.

After his third try at digging into my arm, I found enough courage to ask, "Can I put it in myself?"

I felt like a jerk, but I was desperate. I was also afraid that, if he continued, I would faint, which would have been even more embarrassing. I'd fainted once while on hospital rounds with a prominent internal-medicine physician, who'd thereafter referred to me as "Swooning Suzie."

The resident glanced up at me. Sweat dripped down his forehead and into his eyes.

"No, are you kidding? You'd pass out."

On his fourth vein excavation, I did.

A bit later, still feeling woozy, I met the MRI machine—a new form of humiliation. Scrunching around belly-down on the table, my arms drawn back along my sides, I positioned each breast to fall through its individual peek hole. Then the technician put foam plugs in my ears to deafen the next forty-five minutes of *CLANK... WHAP... WHEEP....*

Even though I knew that the radiologist wouldn't read the images while the machine was running, I imagined him sitting in the control deck, aghast at the huge blur of cancer on the monitor. To ease my mind, I tried counting backwards: "One hundred thousand four hundred and ninety-two...one hundred thousand four hundred and ninety-one..." and then doing multiplication problems: "Seventy-two times thirty-six equals...let's see, six times two is twelve, so that's two, carry the one...." Maybe I should have tried naming state capitals.

The gadolinium contrast shot through the IV and into my body—a refreshing jolt of coolness that offset the machine chamber's warmth. I thought about the gadolinium circulating through my veins and arteries, then reaching my tissues; I imagined which cells were taking it up quickly and which were not, the cancerous separating from the benign on the MRI scan.

Finally the clanking stopped. I was birthed out of the MRI magnet headfirst and face-down. Through my earplugs I heard muffled footsteps, then the technician's words:

"Okay, we're done."

My arms felt numb. I wasn't sure how to raise myself out of the breast peek holes without them.

"We're going to have to image your left breast later," the technician continued. "We could only squeeze in your MRI for the affected side tonight."

I unstuck my face from the mold and looked up at her, spittle plastered to my cheeks. *Affected.* Why couldn't people just say what it was—*cancer*?

Lying on my belly with my head raised, trying to blink clarity into my eyes, I must have looked like a disoriented newborn seal surfacing for air for the first time. My awakening arms prickled on either side of my torso.

Standing between the control deck and me, the technician held a gown open as if she were hanging laundry on the line. I was supposed to get up now. By myself.

I maneuvered myself onto all fours. My bare breasts hung down, but at least they were shielded from the men in the control deck. I hadn't done my radiology rotation yet: I worried that I might run into one of these men in the fall. Awkwardly, I rotated myself to a seated position.

The technician draped the gown over me and ushered me out the door. "They'll contact you with the results."

I was no longer one of "them," the medical people.

Now I was a patient.

In a matter of hours, years of study aimed at carefully constructing myself as a fledgling near-doctor had crumbled away and left me bare. It was ironic: All along I had tried to identify with my patients, to imagine life in their shoes, but now, as a patient myself, I felt ill-prepared for the mounting sense of uncertainty and isolation.

I went back to the dressing room.

Once there, I saw that I'd stuffed my shoes and clothes haphazardly into the cubby, just as I would have done in the surgery locker room before going to an operation. But this was different. Instead of heading into the OR and waiting to be passed the suction wand, an exciting privilege, I would have to wait through an interminable weekend for my MRI results.

I wondered if I would ever hold a suction wand again.

Dressed, I trudged out to the waiting room. The pastel horses were still there, trying to dance out of the painting on the wall.

My friends looked first at the four Band-Aids on my forearm, then up at me for a silent moment.

Then they said, "Let's get you out of here."

About the author: Jessica Les is a graduate of Stanford University School of Medicine and London School of Hygiene and Tropical Medicine. She recently graduated from the Santa Rosa Family Medicine Residency Program, a UCSF affiliate. Her passion for creative nonfiction writing was sparked in Sharon Bray's cancer writing group, and then fanned by a Stanford Medical Scholars Grant. "Affected" is an excerpt from her book, now nearing completion. Jessica's interests also include rambling walks, dogs, making art, sewing inexpertly and, someday, revolutionizing medical training and healthcare delivery. Follow her most recent writing and cancer adventures at www.lesforsuccess.blogspot.com/

Déjà-vu

Justin Sanders
10/1/2010

It looked like the skin of an orange—"peau d'orange," in medspeak. My fellow interns and I had heard about it in medical school; some had even seen it before. As our attending physician undraped Mrs. Durante's breast one sunny morning during our first month as interns, we knew that what we were seeing was bad.

Mrs. Durante wore a hospital gown and a brightly colored head scarf. She looked like a child lying in the bed: small, delicate, demure. Her face was pretty, her voice soft and deep. By contrast, the mass rounding out the side of her right breast bulged aggressively. It was firm to the touch, reddish against her olive skin. When asked, she said it hurt.

Timidly, we interns explored its edges with gentle, over-extended fingers. In Mrs. Durante's armpit we felt a nest of firm nodules—lymph nodes nurtured on a diet of cells growing out of control.

Cancer often hides. Here it was thriving in plain sight. To my surprise, Mrs. Durante had an air of calm detachment, as if the breast we were examining belonged to someone else, as if the pain were not her own.

What became evident that morning was not just the power of cancer but the power of denial. Mrs. Durante knew something was wrong, but had hidden it from her siblings, her husband and three children. She'd watched the lump grow under her skin until the stretching and inflammation became too uncomfortable to ignore. Then she'd sought treatment—for pain. Now, her pain relieved, she lay in bed watching TV, calling her friends and family and never mentioning her cancer.

Her hospital stay was short. We made her an appointment with an oncologist, found her a primary-care doctor and sent her home.

* * * * *

Near the end of that year, I arrived at the hospital one morning to find that Mrs. Durante had returned. Reviewing her chart, I learned that despite several readmissions for pain, she'd never visited the oncologist. She'd gone to her primary-care doctor only for pain medicine and had come to the hospital because it was no longer effective.

I was struck by her appearance: At first glance, she looked much as she had at our first meeting. But her bright, multicolored head scarf and shy smile belied the destruction beneath her hospital gown. Examining her, I saw that her cancerous breast had grown larger, more firm and red. Her neck skin was taut with underlying cancer, her belly swollen with metastases.

Why, I wondered, had she not sought treatment? I found her passivity maddening and puzzling. Our initial treatment plan had formed a simple picture of hope—that medicine could conquer her cancer, could restore her. Her denial—of it, of us—had shattered that hope. I could barely hide my frustration.

"Mrs. Durante," I asked, "what do you think will happen if you don't get treatment for your cancer?"

"I just won't be here anymore," she said.

Could dying be as simple as that? I wondered, then pressed on: "And how do you think that will be for your family?"

She only shrugged, with a glimmer of sadness.

I pleaded with her to meet with the oncologists to discuss her treatment options.

"I just want to get my chemotherapy and go home," she said. "I don't want to have to meet first to talk about it."

In my short career, I'd worked with hospice patients. I'd held people's hands as they took their last breath. But never had I felt so acutely that I was watching someone die right before me. I could practically see her disappearing. I wanted to yell at her to come back to reality.

Finally Mrs. Durante agreed to meet with the oncologists. We arranged to discharge her the next morning directly to her appointment in the oncology clinic, downstairs in the same building. I asked her if I could tell her family her diagnosis, and she consented.

They were shocked—and galvanized: They promised to accompany her to the appointment. Relief flooded through me.

The next morning, Mrs. Durante's brother called: They were late, but en route. Mrs. Durante declined my offer to escort her downstairs, so I told her that her family would meet her at the oncology office. Watching her leave, I wondered if I had done enough to corral her into therapy—or if that was even the right thing to do....

Ten minutes later, her sister called. "We just saw Stella walking away from the hospital. Is she finished with her appointment?"

"No," I said. "Can you get her and bring her back?"

Five minutes later, another call. "She says she went to the appointment already and got her chemotherapy."

"No, she didn't!" I said incredulously. "Can you try to convince her to come back?"

Frantically, I called the oncology clinic to say that Mrs. Durante was on her way. They said they would still see her....

* * * * *

The other day, a young lady of sixteen years walked into my clinic room complaining of a sore throat. Her name was Flora. Tall, thin and shy, she wore a head scarf. She had all the symptoms of strep throat: fever, white patches on her tonsils and swollen, tender lymph nodes. While waiting for the strep test result, I asked her who she lived with.

"My stepfather and my brother and sister. You may have known my mother, Stella Durante? She died in September."

For a moment I caught my breath. The image of a bright head scarf and white, sunlit hospital blankets flashed through my mind.

"I did know your mother," I said. "I'm sorry to hear that she died. How have you been since that happened?"

She shrugged. Suddenly, I felt her mother there in the room.

Despite a normal test result, Flora's symptoms convinced me that she should be treated with antibiotics. Because of her age, or because of my memories of her mother, I feared that she might not complete ten days of pills. I recommended a penicillin shot.

Minutes later, the nurse knocked on my door. Flora was refusing the injection for fear of the pain.

I went to where she sat. Seeing her familiar, somewhat blank expression, I felt a surge of alarm.

"I'm sure it won't hurt as much as you think," I said, mustering authority. "Not as much as the sore throat."

I reflected uncomfortably that I wasn't sure this was true.

"If you absolutely cannot do it, I'll give you the medicine by mouth," I finished. "But I really think you should take the shot."

She finally agreed, and I shut the door behind me, praying she wouldn't change her mind.

Later, while writing my notes, I felt the adrenaline rush fading away. A penicillin injection had never felt so urgent. An image of Flora's mother came to mind. She was walking down the street, untreated. I didn't ever want that to happen again.

About the author: *Justin Sanders is a family physician currently based in Northampton, MA. "I've always loved writing as a means of expression, but I sharpened my pen by writing letters to a long-distance love, to whom I've been married now for going on two years. When not working, I like looking at contemporary paintings, cooking pizza and reading* The New Yorker.*"*

going blind

Kirstyn Smith
10/8/2010

I still dream Crayola: Scarlet, cherry, candy apple;
Zeus' breath, Antiguan shallows, Atlantic turmoil, August twilight;
Green sings lime, martini olive, cypress, spring meadow, life.
When I woke up this morning, I wanted to turn over.
Of course, you feel the same way.

I had a dream about cleaning my fingernails. I had this beautiful, shiny silver file and I
could see the brown of the dirt. Peach, compost, and ivory. Each nail suffered caked mud
beneath the many split layers, great time and precision to extract the telling debris.
I worked to carve out the dirt, to rid my hands of the everyday work mess that drives my
soul and gossips my menial livelihood.

And I wish I could say that there was a dramatic culmination to my metaphorical dream. But I can't. There wasn't.

I opened my eyes to see the plain old brown-grey dark
that has been my life since the birth of my last child, the blindness that has coated my
every movement, every thought, every intention
since before I could awaken to color and breathe.

Most days, I do not roll over. I don't attempt to recapture the lost.
I trust my doctors to dream their colorful dreams for me.

I throw off the sheets and groan the same thing you do,
"Good morning. It's time to get up."

And we all roll out of our lovely dreams and begin this day.
But I have no crayons.

About the poet: *Kirstyn Smith is an English educator, amateur writer, gardener and cook. She is also a mom and community volunteer. Her writing has appeared in* The Cornell Daily Sun *and in* Mercedes *magazine, but most often in letters to her children from Santa Claus and the Tooth Fairy. Kirstyn has been losing her vision and gaining her insight since the age of eight, when she was diagnosed with a chronic degenerative eye condition. Since the total loss of her sight, she has found solace in the written word, the photographs it creates in the mind's eye and the nuance of shifting perspectives that it engenders in readers.*

About the poem: *"This piece began as a Stephen Moss–inspired fifty-five-word story, a concept to which I was introduced by a dear friend who is a physician and fellow reader/writer. The fifty-five-word draft felt more like an unused coloring sheet than a complete picture. As the weather changed in the mid-Atlantic region this fall, the colors that faded from the landscape ignited my memory and fueled my fingers to type the hues and textures between the black lines in this version of the story."*

toothache

Majid Khan
10/15/2010

I always look forward to meeting new patients—and I confess that I have a particular fondness for young patients. They are, you see, at the point in their lives where everything is possible. It's possible to have fun when other people might feel upset, possible to enjoy oneself on Friday night after a hard week of work (or study) rather than complaining about being too tired. I love sharing in their dreams, their joys, their fun and their excitement.

My first patient this morning is thirty-year-old Kieran. We've never met; I wonder what she's been up to, and if she's planning any adventures. I'm looking forward to chatting, to exploring the "biopsychosocial" aspect of her medical complaint, as I keep urging my own students to do.

If only I didn't have this damn toothache.

It's my right lower wisdom tooth, I think. It's been throbbing on and off for the past few weeks. I've been chewing on my left side in the hope that the ache will just go away, but it hasn't; it catches me unawares whenever I absent-mindedly chew on the right.

Kieran, smiling and energetic even at this early hour, tells me her medical troubles—mainly an intermittent headache. She describes it vividly, with such dramatic passion that I'm swept away: I almost feel that *I'm* the one who's experiencing the headache.

Okay, it's time to explore her social history. After some discussion, we agree that her headaches are most likely tension-related. We arrange a return visit in one week, and I give her some general stress-reduction advice.

As we talk, I learn that she's a dentist.

Now, there's a bit of luck! I ask her to take a look at my tooth, which she readily agrees to do.

Rising from her chair, she asks for a tongue depressor and a flashlight.

"Do you have thirty-two teeth?" she begins.

"Er...I don't know," I answer, thinking that this sounds like rather a lot of teeth for one mouth.

"Umm..." she says, scanning my molars, "You have a cavity. You may need RCT."

Randomized controlled trial? I think.

"But I've only got a bit of toothache," I say. My face shows my confusion.

"Root canal treatment," she says.

"Oh."

I get up, thanking her for her help. But something has been bugging me, and I feel I just have to ask.

"Where do these teeth come from?" I say, pointing to my bottom molars.

"From the mandible," she answers.

"So this tooth"—I point to the throbbing molar—"is in fact the mandible in a different version?"

"Kind of."

"Would it be more accurate to say that the tooth *is* the mandible?"

"No," she says firmly. "It's a tooth."

"But that part of the mandible *becomes* the tooth?"

"Yes."

"I see."

I thank her, and we say goodbye.

I feel ever so slightly satisfied. But hang on a minute—the mandible comes from whatever it came from, which means that the mandible *isn't* the mandible, it's a different version of whatever gave rise to it. In this sense, it would seem that everything is the same as everything else. It's all just different versions of a single "oneness."

When my tooth is hurting, I observe, my right hand stops what it's engaged in—it puts the pen to one side and lifts up compassionately to soothe my aching tooth. Even my mind stops whatever it's engaged in and concentrates instead on how to relieve the discomfort. The pain is in my tooth, not in my arm, my eye or my mind—yet this entire body feels the pain.

I wonder if a similar oneness applies to me in relation to another suffering human. Can his or her suffering also be mine? Are we all just different versions of the same oneness? Do we depend on one another in this way for our very existence?

Tomorrow I'm flying to New York for a mindfulness retreat; I'll ask the chaps there what they think about it.

Packing my bags at home that night, I cast furtive glances at my mother, seated across the room. This is the third time I'm traveling this year, and I know she disapproves of my going away. But such is the life of a Pakistani man in the UK: Mum's opinions are still important.

"Where are you going?" she asks.

"America."

"Why?"

Attempting to translate "a three-day retreat in mindful medical practice" into Pashto would be ridiculous, so I answer simply, "For a meeting."

I wait for the flaring of the nostrils, the disgusted sweeping away of the face. Quickly, I change the subject.

"What do you want me to bring you back?"

"Whatever—do they do head scarves there?"

"I'm sure they will. It's America, after all."

Her mood lightens, and because of this, so does mine. It is as though her mood has *become* mine.

"Shall I make you some tea?" she asks.

"Okay," I reply.

The teabags, water, sweetener, cinnamon and milk miraculously become the tea, which the two of us sip together, sitting cross-legged on the floor as is the Pakistani custom and talking about the good old days—my long-deceased father, what it was like in the village where they grew up.

I reflect on the utterly incomprehensible number of conditions that have led to this moment. Somehow, all of these conditions have given rise to this mother and son, sitting together on the floor of this front room. We are not separate from these conditions; we result from them.

Suddenly I remember Kieran. I wonder how her headache is. It's as though Kieran's pain is mine, because it could be no other way.

Soon, though, my thoughts are interrupted.

"Majid," says mum.

"Yes?" I ask quietly, like a father speaking comfortingly to a two-year-old.

"My tooth has been hurting me...."

About the author: *Majid Khan is a general practitioner in Birmingham, UK. He teaches communication skills at Warwick Medical School, where he is also in the process of setting up a course in mindful medical practice and becoming a mindfulness teacher. Another of his stories has appeared in* BJGP: The British Journal of General Practice. *Other personal interests include Buddhism, spirituality and mathematics. He dedicates this story:*

To my books, for teaching me much,
To my teachers, for teaching me much more,
To my patients, for teaching me everything.

Adam

Genevieve Yates
10/22/2010

I tried to focus on the chart in front of me, but it may as well have been written in Russian. I'd been awake for thirty-two hours, and my brain, thick with fatigue, refused to cooperate. I knew I shouldn't be working, but I was too proud, too stubborn, too *something* to admit that I wasn't coping.

On the first day of my neurosurgical rotation, the resident I was replacing had told me, "Ten-to-fourteen-hour days, twelve days on, two days off. Say goodbye to your life for the next three months!"

I was prepared for the long hours, endless paperwork and ward-round humiliations. I expected that it might be necessary to take a leave of absence from my personal life. What I didn't expect was that my personal and working lives would collide headlong.

As I sat there, not writing up ward-round notes, my boyfriend, Adam, lay across the hall in the neurosurgical ICU. Twenty-four hours earlier, he'd had a tumor removed from the back of his brain.

We'd met in the med-school library when I was a final-year medical student: Waiting in line for the photocopier, we'd struck up a conversation. Adam had just been diagnosed with testicular cancer; he was reading up on the disease. His warm brown eyes and infectious smile attracted me instantly, and his humor and glass-half-full attitude completed the job. We went out for coffee that evening and soon became inseparable.

Adam was a country boy from the outback, with a passion for competitive sheep shearing. He had a keen intelligence and although, or perhaps because, he hadn't attended college, he felt a deep connection with and appreciation of the natural world.

For several months after his initial treatment had finished, Adam and I enjoyed a fairytale romance. In remission, and with a 98 percent chance of cure, my one-testicled Prince Charming introduced me to many of the joys I'd been too preoccupied to notice.

One Saturday morning he said, "This weather is so good, it would be criminal to waste it. Are you up for a weekend down the Coast?" Before I had time to even consider, I found myself picnicking with Adam in the rainforest, luxuriating in a spa and walking together along the beach by moonlight, gazing up at the stars.

Those heady, carefree days didn't last. Ten months after his initial diagnosis, as I was working as a neurosurgical intern, Adam had a seizure. He ended up on my ward, diagnosed with an occipital lobe metastasis: the cancer had spread to his brain. (True to form, he joked that growing a brain tumor showed just how far he'd go to see the woman he loved.) For obvious reasons I wasn't his doctor, but his being on my ward gave us many opportunities to sneak in some time together—the situation's only silver lining.

The nurse's voice penetrated my mental fog.

"Adam's back from the ICU. Apparently he just got up and left." She shook her head affectionately. "That boy is something else."

As I approached Adam's bedside, he smiled broadly, looking pale but lively, the bandages around his head somewhat askew.

"What's this I hear about your walking out of intensive care?" I asked with mock sternness.

"That place is creepy—full of really sick people. I figured it would be much better to be back on this ward. I knew a bed was being a held for me, so I grabbed my IV stand and walked here."

"But you had brain surgery yesterday!" I protested.

"Yeah, so?"

Two days later, Adam turned up on my doorstep bearing gifts. He'd discharged himself from the hospital: "I didn't want to be stuck in there when you were having your only day off in two weeks."

He seemed invincible. His inspiration was Lance Armstrong, who'd survived a diagnosis of testicular cancer with metastases in the brain, abdomen and lungs. Soon, however, it became clear that, for Adam, a cure was not going to be possible. Despite surgery and several weeks of radiation therapy, his tumor markers steadily increased. In a matter of months, new tumors were visible on his CT scan. His doctors encouraged further treatment.

They removed almost all of his occipital lobes, which drastically reduced his visual fields, leaving him only a tiny, blurry window through which he viewed the external world. When the tumors appeared elsewhere in his brain, they gave him more radiotherapy and chemotherapy. I felt they knew, deep down, that they were rapidly losing the battle, but still they peddled hope like a drug to my vulnerable Adam, saying, "It's unlikely to work, but it's possible. We can try." Adam had always said that he didn't want to prolong the inevitable, but when push came to shove, offered even a remote chance of cure, he couldn't say no.

As a result, Adam did not have a good death. He spent most of the final weeks of his life in an acute care ward being subjected to unpleasant treatment regimes. Although I felt powerless to do anything, I still regret letting this happen.

In medical school, they'd told us that we would learn more from real-life patients than from lectures and textbooks. Especially from patients we can't fix. Patients who die. They were right. What they didn't say was that watching a loved one struggle against and ultimately lose the battle with an incurable disease would teach us things that years of medical training never could.

Adam gave me a very special gift. Through our journey together, I learned that treating cancer is about so much more than trying to find a cure. It's about more than whether the patient lives or dies. It's about how whatever life left is lived, and ultimately, how one dies.

I learned, too, that a patient's death is not the end of the story. Today, in my own practice, I try hard to actively involve my palliative patients' family and friends, and I continue to offer them care and support even after their loved one has died.

Adam has made me a better person—and a better doctor. I owe him so much. I can't pay it back, but I am trying to pay it forward.

I'm sure he'd be pleased.

In loving memory of Adam Humphries, March 14, 1978–November 12, 2000

About the author: Genevieve Yates is a family physician and medical educator from Australia who is passionate about putting creativity into medicine and medicine into creativity. A columnist for the medical newspaper Australian Doctor, *she has also had several short stories published, a short film produced and five plays staged. Her first novel,* Silver Linings, *was published in 2011. She's also worked in film and TV and has performed in plays, musicals and stand-up comedy. Genevieve teaches violin, plays piano, sings and plays in two orchestras. In 2010, she received the Arts and Health Australia Awards for Excellence: Medical Humanities and Education Award. "I use film, theater and music in my teaching and find that medicine inspires and complements my writing and vice-versa."*

Life of the party

Veneta Masson
10/29/2010

By ones and twos
we drift up to the bedroom—
the women of the family—
leaving the men to mutter
and churn downstairs.
This is women's work,
choosing a burial outfit.
We have a list from the mortuary:
bring underthings
no shoes

Soberly we peer into the closet
slide open drawers
touch, handle, inhale.
Ah, I was with her when she bought this...
Remember the time?
What about a hat?
Oh yes, she loved hats!
No, not that! someone laughs.
Someone laughed!

We begin to try on, critique.
Soon the room is festooned
with strewn fashion.
We turn giddy, intimate
acquisitive—
a raucous sisterhood.

Next day some are subdued.
We got carried away...
Maybe it wasn't right...
And yet at the time—
in the moment—
and hadn't she been
the life of the party?

About the poet: *Veneta Masson is a nurse and poet living in Washington, DC. Her work is often inspired by her clinical experiences, or, as in the case of this poem, by a family caregiver. You can find more of her work at* www.sagefemmepress.com.

About the poem: *"Who hasn't had the shocking experience of laughing in the face of tragedy? At first it feels wrong wrong wrong. But what a gift it can be—giving us the strength to gather ourselves and carry on. I'll never forget that evening in my sister's bedroom, the fragile hilarity that erupted and the doubts that arose the next day. This is the slice of life I've tried to portray in my poem."*

Bruised

Eileen M.K. Bobek
11/5/2010

The year after I finished my emergency-medicine residency, I had all four of my wisdom teeth pulled.

Afterwards, I looked as if I had taken several punches to my face. My jaw was swollen, my skin a cornucopia of muddied blues, purples, greens, yellows and reds. If people didn't know better, I told my husband with a laugh, they might think that I'd been beaten.

It took weeks for the swelling and discoloration to resolve. I went about my life, aware of both my face and people's responses to it. Their pitying, uncomfortable, sometimes disgusted expressions told me what they were thinking: I was being abused. But nobody ever asked me how I was, how it had happened or even if it hurt.

"I can't believe it!" I'd rail to my husband. "Not one person has asked. Not one!"

It wasn't long before my disbelief gave way to resentment. I started testing people. When our eyes met, I'd refuse to look away, silently daring them to ignore my face. Sometimes I'd relent and reveal that I'd had some teeth pulled. An expression of relief, tinged with lingering suspicion, would wash over their faces. But their nervous laughter and the tension that evaporated from their shoulders told me that their relief was not for me; i]t was for them. I'd absolved them of the responsibility of asking.

Most of the time, I said nothing, letting the weight of their silence hang in the air between us. Their guilt made me feel certain that I would never be silent.

* * * * *

I still don't know her name.

I saw her only at my six-year-old son's weekly T-ball games, five years ago. She and her two young sons had the benign, nondescript look of the families advertised in picture frames—all feathery light-brown hair and creamy skin.

Her husband dressed in oxford shirts and business slacks, a beeper clinging to his belt. He was a grim-faced Ken doll—clean-shaven, with immobile sandy brown hair and a mouth locked in a thin line.

Once, she and I chatted on the sidelines as our three-year-old boys played together alongside the baseball field. At some point, her son picked up the Styrofoam cup next to her and took a drink from the straw. I saw her husband's face darken, his body stiffen. He strode from the first base line where he'd been coaching and snatched the cup from his son's hands, slamming it into the garbage before returning to first base.

The boy retreated to his mother's lap, leaning his body into hers. As she dipped her head over his, she said, "You know you shouldn't take Daddy's drink."

I thought I saw her glance at me through the curtain of her hair. We never spoke again.

I don't remember seeing her again until the end of the season. She was sitting on the ground, handing out drinks and snacks to the players. As they swarmed around her like bees, I walked over with my sons. She looked up.

The wind whipped back her hair to reveal a black eye.

She'd made no attempt to hide it; she wasn't wearing makeup or sunglasses. Her defiant expression mirrored my own of so many years before; she was testing me.

I imagined us in the ER—she sheltered within the walls of a patient room, me sheltered within my white doctor's coat, freed from my fear and embarrassment and empowered to ask her the question on my lips. If she denied being beaten and got indignant or angry, I could retreat into my role: *It's my responsibility to ask.* If she admitted it, I could offer her help—social work, counseling, a safe house, *something*. But without my coat, there on our sons' playing field, I felt stripped of my power and authority—a not-so-super hero, crippled without her costume.

I said nothing. *There are too many children around,* I told myself. *This is not the time.*

We held each other's gaze for a few seconds; then she turned away.

Instantly, I knew that I'd made a mistake—but the moment was lost. I reassured myself that I would have another chance; I'd see her after the game, at the nearby ice cream store where they handed out the trophies.

When I didn't see her there, I approached another mother.

"Do you know the woman at the game who was handing out snacks? She had a black eye. I was wondering if she's all right."

She started, darting her eyes away as she stammered, "I...uh...no...I don't know...I see my son." She hurried past me, trailing a string of unintelligible words.

It was then that I turned and saw her husband and two sons sitting in a booth ten feet away, eating their ice-cream cones in silence. As my son received his trophy, I scanned the entrance for her, willing her to show up and come through the glass doors; she never appeared.

I still think of her sometimes. I don't know whether her black eye happened by accident or intention. Remembering her husband's angry response to his young son, I think I know—but still I want to deny.

I recall my own bruised and swollen face and my disbelief that so many people so easily let me go without a word of concern or curiosity. I imagine how alone I would have felt if the unspoken suspicion on their faces had been justified. And I remember her face—defiant, bare of makeup, as if she were testing us, hoping someone might ask. If I had asked, maybe she would have said it was nothing. Maybe she would have lied but also taken comfort in knowing that someone had dared enough, cared enough to ask.

That moment—the wind blowing back her hair, her eyes meeting mine—replays in my mind like an endless loop. I think of all the things I could have said. *Are you okay? How did it happen? Does it hurt?*

I want to believe that I would never make the same mistake again—that my fear would never again overwhelm my compassion and decency.

I can't help but think that's why she didn't show up later. She had taken a chance on us, and we'd all failed her. *I* had failed her. I'd had my one chance—and let it slip away.

About the author: *Eileen M. K. Bobek is a former emergency-medicine physician. Her work has also been published in* hip Mama *magazine.*

girl talk

Warren Holleman
11/12/2010

"I got pregnant. Quit sports, quit school. Quit all my dreams."

Brenda looks fit and handsome, despite the scar running down the middle of her face. At six feet tall, she commands respect, even though her sweet, high-pitched voice belies her imposing physique.

We are sitting in a circle: Brenda, six other women and me. Most are in their thirties and forties, and in their fourth or fifth month of sobriety. They look professional in the suits they've assembled from the donations closet of our inner-city recovery center.

No one is surprised when Brenda says that, twenty years ago, she trained for the U.S. Olympic volleyball team.

"Did you ever compete again?" someone asks.

"Nope."

"Why not?"

Brenda shakes her head. The group gives her a moment to think about it, to grieve the loss.

"Later, I took up tennis. I was pretty good! Won lots of tournaments. You know, local stuff."

Brenda pauses, then continues. "The people I played with, they were doctors, lawyers, people like that. Which was kinda cool. But this was the Eighties, and everybody was using powder cocaine. You know what I mean?"

The older ladies do know what she means. They nod and cast glances around the room.

"And something else happened." She takes a deep breath. "I met this man."

Everybody perks up. They're hoping against hope for a good love story.

"And you fell in love with him?"

"Oh no! I ain't THAT crazy."

"Falling in love ain't crazy."

"He was seventy years old. I was twenty-five."

"Yeah. So why are you telling us about him?"

"Because I married him."

"You *what*?"

"Girl. He had money and a four-bedroom house. That sounded soooo good."

"Wow!"

More nods and smiles and glances. "And?"

"And what?"

"Was it worth it?"

"Hell no!"

"Four bedrooms is a lot of real estate."

"He was this LITTLE man."

"So?"

"This was his fifth marriage."

"I could put up with a lot for four bedrooms."

"He was a sicko."

"Girl! What could he do to YOU?"

A pregnant pause. Brenda starts to look angry. "He could beat me. He could belittle me."

"I don't see how."

"I was fucked up. Hooked on his money. Hooked on his cocaine."

Brenda looks around the room, then up. She talks to the ceiling: "After I left him, I couldn't afford no more powder. So then I did something REALLY stupid. I got hooked on crack."

She lowers her gaze. "I told you I was fucked up."

The ladies begin commiserating: "Like WE wasn't fucked up? At least you knew where to come to for help."

"Sure! It only took me fifteen years!"

She's angry, mostly at herself, but also at the others for trying to cheer her up. "I wasted fifteen years."

She stops talking, but no one dares speak. The only sound is her breathing. She's trying to figure out some way to redeem those fifteen years.

Suddenly, she perks up. "Hey! Maybe you ladies can learn from my mistakes."

One by one, they respond: "We're listenin'." "We're learnin'." "You've helped me see somethin'."

I'm supposed to be leading this group, but so far I haven't said a word. All the ladies appear engaged.

Except for Sabrina.

Sabrina is eighteen. She's the youngest, the group mascot. Unlike the others, she's wearing a tight skirt and showing cleavage. A few weeks ago, when the group began, she told us that she's tired of living on the street. This morning she's been quiet, taking it all in. Finally, she speaks.

"You said 'sicko'—your husband was a sicko. What do you mean, sicko?"

"He had a lead pipe. He covered it with rubber padding. He just liked to walk around holding it in his hand."

"Whoa," says one of the ladies.

"Hmm," says another.

"He didn't scare me, 'cause I was a LOT bigger than him."

"So what's the problem?" Sabrina asks.

"He hit me—hard. He put me in a coma. For five days they didn't know if I'd wake up. And what would be left if I did."

Silence.

"You do see the scar—right?" It was wide as a pencil and ran from her hairline to halfway down her nose.

Finally, they begin talking: "I always wondered how you got that." "I was afraid to say anything." One woman reaches out to take Brenda's hands: "Oh baby, he hurt you bad."

"I was the type..." Brenda's eyes begin to water. Someone hands her a tissue. "I had to learn my lesson the hard way."

A quiet understanding fills the air. The other women have been there them-selves. We let it all sink in.

I'm the one who breaks the silence. "You said you learned your lesson the hard way. From the feeling in here, I'm sensing that this was a really impor-tant lesson." Nods of recognition around the room. "How would you put it into words?"

"Never marry a man for his money—it ain't worth it," says Brenda. "If ever it was worth it, it would have been with this man. He had a ton of money."

The chorus responds: "I hear you, darlin'." "You sure got that right." "Oh yeah." Then from the other side of the circle: "Amen. We love you, baby."

Except for Sabrina, everyone has spoken. All eyes turn to her as she stirs to attention.

"This man, is he still alive?"

Brenda puts her hand on Sabrina's shoulder and leans forward to face her, nearly touching forehead to forehead. "Honey, I don't think he'll EVER die!"

The other women laugh and shake their heads. I relax, thinking that's the end of the session.

But Sabrina has more to say.

"Hey! Tell me where he is. I'd like that money."

I sure didn't see that coming. I want to be her father—to tell her, "Stop look-ing for quick fixes! Don't depend on men to take care of you!" and to remind her of all the life lessons she's heard in this circle so far. Which, of course, would only drive her in the other direction.

Fortunately, I'm too stunned to speak.

With sad smiles and shrugs, the older women give Sabrina the feedback she needs: a warning against following in Brenda's footsteps, plus resignation at her lack of insight.

Although Sabrina clearly doesn't want to seem like she's taking their advice, I know that it's registered. Even if she doesn't say so, she'll think about it. I hope she'll let it sink in—either now or after her next mistake.

It's nine o'clock, time for our break.

And, feeling as wrung out as I do between my concern for Brenda and my anxiety for Sabrina, I need one.

About the author: *Warren Holleman is a family therapist who worked for many years in a recovery program for homeless women. He currently serves as professor of behavioral science and director of the faculty health and well-being program at the University of Texas-MD Anderson Cancer Center. He is also co-editor of the textbook* Fundamentals of Clinical Practice, *a textbook for medical students, and an award-winning playwright. "I grew up in eastern North Carolina, pretending not to listen to the rambling stories my father and uncles told me. Then I moved to Texas and found my way into a profession whose primary job requirement is...listening to stories. And now I enjoy telling stories—those of my elders, and those of my own—to all comers, whether they listen, pretend to listen or pretend not to."*

semi-private room

Jan Jahner
11/19/2010

Sometimes nectar appears
when stories intersect:

> I walk into the room
> rearrange the bed-table
> and push the pole with its bulging bladder sideways
> for a closer look.

> Her thinness triples the size of the bed
> but her father, with his anxious chatter
> feels strangely like my own
> and her resolve, that tense control
> has a familiar edge.

> It feels like all the calories she's ever counted
> and all the sweet things resisted for the last eleven years
> have aligned as a taut shield
> protecting that juicy place that hasn't ripened,
> urged too early to carry her family through chaos:
> > after all, her mother was dying of cancer
> > after all, mine couldn't manage mental illness
> > after all, aren't fathers helpless in these things?

> The electrolyte imbalance that nearly took her life
> and the nurturance imbalance that emptied
> her adolescent pockets of all the in-free tickets,
> lie tangled with the feeding tube she never wanted
> while she talks and I listen, my beeper ignored.

> Our connection becomes a spoon
> with its delicate curve
> Starting the good-byes, I hand her my card
> she reads through the menu
> departing, I feel the full moon
> rising in my chest.

__About the poet:__ Navigating emergency, hospice and palliative-care nursing has provided Jan Jahner with rich and rewarding relationships for the last twenty-eight years. Currently, she is the palliative-care coordinator at Christus St. Vincent's Hospital in Santa Fe, NM. In 2007 she received the National Hospice Foundation's Project on Death in America Nursing Leadership Award for her work in rural communities. Along with expressive writing, Jan enjoys pretty much anything connected with the great outdoors, her children and grandchildren and spiritual inquiry; as a writer, she focuses on the feelings or phrases that emerge while sitting at a patient's bedside or conversing with colleagues about patient care.

__About the poem:__ "Most of my poems emerge from the specific residue of a clinical encounter that wants more time and attention. I enjoy sorting out the interconnected elements of the parallel process involved in giving and receiving care. The young woman in this poem hoped to become a nurse."

tea and daisies

Amy Cooper Rodriguez
11/26/2010

It's been almost ten years since Esther died, and I still think of her almost every day. I was her physical therapist at a rehabilitation hospital. My patients had many different diagnoses—head injury, stroke, multiple sclerosis, hip or knee replacements. I was in my early twenties. I thought that if I tried hard enough, I could help everyone. And often, I could.

* * * * *

"What are you going to do to me?" Esther asked, looking up from her hospital chair.

I laughed and pulled up a chair. "I'm Amy, your physical therapist. I'm not going to do anything to you. I'm here to help you get back to doing things you miss."

Esther smoothed her long skirt over her plump legs, then pushed her glasses up on her nose. "I just want to go home and be able to do things for myself."

"All right. We'll work together to get you stronger and back home," I said confidently.

Nobody could tell why Esther felt weak. Doctors said maybe it was old age (she was eighty), arthritis or a vitamin deficiency. She had to use her hands to lift her legs in and out of bed. It took her five tries to get up out of her chair.

Over the next two weeks, I worked with Esther every day. A former English teacher, she believed she had a reputation to maintain. Before we left for the gym, she'd brush her soft, gray curls and freshen up her lipstick. She exercised wearing a dress, nylons and shoes with little heels.

Esther was private and proud, and only slowly revealed herself. She grew daisies, drank Earl Grey tea and loved a good crossword puzzle. I felt I knew her. I come from a long line of reticent Yankees, including my adored grandmother. I was used to talking about tea and daisies instead of feelings. Even at twenty-five, I connected with Esther more than I did with most people my age.

"What's happening with that boyfriend of yours? How's your crazy land-lord?" she'd ask, deflecting my questions.

One day, I told her that her daughter had called.

"What the heck is she worried about?" Esther grumbled, then went on, "She worries about me. We've really only had each other. My husband and son died in a car accident when she was little. It's been hard on her."

"Oh, Esther," I said, putting a hand on her shoulder. "I'm so, so sorry."

Every day, the nurses gave me a report: "Amy, Esther's stumbling around her room by herself! She's not safe. You need to talk to her. She makes her own bed, for Pete's sake!"

But how could I scold her when I admired her stubbornness? And when I nagged her, "Esther, are you kidding me? Where's your walker?" it was to no avail. I was the therapist, but we both knew she was the boss.

After two weeks of therapy, Esther was strong enough to go home. A month later, though, she was back after a fall. I hurried to her room and hugged her.

"Silly me, I just had to see you again," she laughed. But I could see that she was weaker than before.

I encouraged her to have breakfast with the other patients. "It'll be great! You'll meet other nice people. You might even get some good food!" Then I saw her push her glasses aside to wipe away tears.

"I can't do it," she whispered. "I hate choking in front of people."

Why was she choking?

I planned a home evaluation. Esther wore a floral dress, bright pink lipstick and heels. "I can't wait to make you some tea," she said. But by the time we got to her house, she could barely move. She couldn't turn the key. She couldn't step over the threshold. Trying to look like I didn't notice, I helped her through the door and into a chair.

Though neither of us said so, we both knew this was the last time she would be in her home. I let her shuffle around the kitchen, clumsily fill the teapot and wrestle with the china teacups. Like two old friends, we sat and sipped tea together.

Back at the hospital, her doctors had gathered, shaking their heads. Tests had confirmed their quietly mounting suspicion that Esther had ALS—Lou Gehrig's disease. Their guess was that she had a year or two to live.

As they told Esther about the advances in treatment and gave her brochures, I hugged her slumped shoulders. The dove on the brochure made death look so hopeful.

Then they tried to place a breathing mask on her face. She shook her head: "No."

I wanted her to put it on, but realized it wasn't my decision.

The next morning, I went to Esther's room before taking off my coat. She lay on a stretcher, the mask now covering her face. She was being transferred to the regional hospital, no longer a candidate for rehab.

As the EMTs busily strapped her in, her eyes pleaded with me to understand. I laid my head on her shoulder.

"I love you," I said. "Do what you need to do. It's okay." Tears rolled from my eyes.

"Is she your mom?" asked an EMT. I shook my head, and they rolled her away.

After work, as the sky turned pink, I drove down Route 95 to Esther's new hospital, where I asked a smiling lady at the front desk where I could find Esther. The woman looked at her computer and frowned.

"I have her name, but I don't know where she is." She turned the console and pointed. "Esther C. Status: D."

Esther's eyes had told me. She'd been through enough. She no longer wanted to fight. She didn't want to live with breathing machines and feeding tubes, waiting for another day of decline. She wanted to leave on her own terms.

I'd been fortunate to have twenty-five years of innocence, believing that I had the power to fix problems and take away pain. With Esther, I learned the harsh reality: I can't always do that.

What I can do is listen to what my patients want—even if it means feeling uncomfortable and helpless. Sometimes I need to sit quietly and let them get their own lipstick, pour their own tea or refuse medical care.

Esther also showed me that it's okay to cry with my patients, and that sometimes there are no words. And while she could see the old soul in me, I could see the young soul in her—the one who once must have been so effervescent.

It's been ten years, and I still think about Esther. I hope that somewhere she's wearing her sassiest shoes and her brightest lipstick. More than anything, I hope she knows how much she taught me.

About the author: Amy Cooper Rodriguez is a writer and mom who has worked as a physical therapist and teacher. In these jobs, she has been honored to hear people's stories. She blogs about parenting and mental health for Psychology Today *at* http://www.psychologytoday.com/blog/parenting-the-blues. *She also writes for a number of other magazines, and her published works can be found on her Web site,* www.parentingontheloose.com.

Lost in the Numbers

Don Stewart
12/3/2010

A nurse entered the operating room. Her eyes—the only part of her face visible above her surgical mask—held a look of mild distress. She stood quietly until the surgeon noticed her.

"What is it?" he said.

"It's your patient in 208, Doctor. His pressure is 82."

"Systolic?"

"Yes, Doctor."

The nurse was referring to Mr. Johnson. The previous week, we'd removed a small tumor from his lung without difficulty—and, until now, without complications. He'd been transferred out of Intensive Care to the main surgical floor, and that very morning we had removed the last drainage tubes from his chest. He was scheduled to go home the next day.

Now his blood pressure was plummeting.

"Doctor Stewart, break scrub and go see what's going on. Nurse, grab that retractor."

Grateful for the break in a mind-numbing routine (as a surgical intern, my job in the OR was to stand for hours, holding the incision open as the surgeons worked), I stepped away from the table and out of the room, removing my sterile gown and gloves along the way. Running up the stairs to the second floor (surgical residents, like the military, take the steps two at a time), I hurried toward Mr. Johnson's room.

Normal resting blood pressure is 120 over 80. The higher number reflects the force of blood within the vessels during heartbeats; the lower number tells how much pressure remains between beats. Mr. Johnson's higher number had just fallen to two-thirds its normal value. His lower number was undetectable. This sudden loss of pressure meant that there could be a leak somewhere—a big one. This man might be bleeding to death internally.

There was no time to waste.

As I rushed along the hallway to his room, I thought through the possibilities: The staples in our patient's lung might have given way. Part of his wound might have ruptured, leaking blood into his chest. We might have ripped a small artery while removing his chest tubes that morning. He could be suffering from a sudden, overwhelming infection or an allergic reaction to a medication. The stress of the surgery might have caused bleeding ulcers in his stomach, or a heart attack. Whatever the cause, I expected to find him in bad shape—pale, light-headed, possibly unresponsive.

I tried to plan ahead: Push IV fluids. Order blood transfusions. Get an EKG—and a chest x-ray. Would he need emergency surgery? Gastric endoscopy? Cardiac consult? Stool sample? Just weeks out of medical school, I felt all these tests and treatments bouncing around in my head like numbers in a lottery. Somewhere in the mix, I felt certain, lurked the *real* problem—the one I hadn't thought of, the one I might continue to miss until after my patient had expired.

First things first: Examine the incisions, listen to the patient's chest. Check his temperature. See if his blood pressure was still falling.

I rounded the corner to room 208, knocked and entered, then stopped short, shocked.

Mr. Johnson was sitting up in bed, smiling and chatting with his wife. His skin was pink. His lips were rosy red. His eyes were clear.

He said he was feeling fine. I believed him.

"No light-headedness?"

"No."

"No new pain or distress?"

"None."

"No complaints at all?"

"No—except that the nurse keeps bothering me about taking my blood pressure."

Right on cue, the RN rolled in a portable blood-pressure cuff. "Doctor, I'm glad you're here. This patient's pressure has been hovering around 80," she said. "Something needs to be done—quickly."

I hesitated, confused, trying to reconcile her concern with Mr. Johnson's obvious state of health.

"Check it yourself!" she said, thrusting the apparatus toward me.

Just then an orderly (now they're called nursing assistants) walked in. He gave the nurse a sideways glance, then said, "That cuff's readings have been all over the map. It needs to be fixed—or thrown out."

Utter relief washed over me. The long list of possible diagnoses, complications and treatments wafted out of my mind, replaced by an enveloping sense of solace and calm—a rare experience for a surgical intern.

I bade Mr. Johnson goodbye and told him that we'd return in a few hours for evening rounds.

Back in the OR, I gave my report.

"The patient was fine."

"What was his blood pressure?" asked the surgeon.

"I didn't check it. The cuff was broken, and there wasn't another one available."

"What did his lungs sound like?"

"I didn't listen to them. He was sitting up and talking, with no shortness of breath, no anxiety, no distress."

"How was his wound?"

"I didn't see it. The nurse had just applied a fresh dressing; she said that it looked fine."

"What was his temperature?"

"I glanced at his chart. His temp was normal a half-hour ago, and it's been stable for days."

The surgeon looked up at me sharply, his eyes blazing over the top of his mask. His reaction shook the room.

"You *didn't* examine your patient? You *didn't* check his blood pressure? *You didn't even take his temperature?!*"

My neglect and incompetence, he told me, could mean the end of my patient—and maybe my medical career. I was to return to the floor immediately, conduct the indicated tests and report back in short order.

Of course I complied—only this time, I took the stairs one at a time.

A thorough exam revealed that the patient's blood pressure was normal. His wound looked fine. His lungs were clear. His temperature was 98.6...

My initial assessment was confirmed to the satisfaction of the floor nurse and the attending surgeon. But the importance of my being able to make that assessment, based on my own powers of observation and clinical judgment, had seemingly gotten lost in the numbers.

The surgeon was right about one thing. In the new era of defensive medicine, with its increasing demand for objective data, the kind of medicine I'd imagined practicing was quickly slipping into history. In every sense, my days as a doctor were numbered.

———————

About the author: Don Stewart earned his bachelor's degree in biology and art at Birmingham-Southern College, where he enrolled in art classes as a change of pace from his premedical studies. Don continued to pursue artistic interests as a hobby at the University of Alabama School of Medicine and during a surgical internship at the Mayo Clinic, where he received awards for both short fiction and poetry and published his first two composite drawings. He has since worked as an artist and writer at the DS Art Studio, where he continues to refine his signature style of visual humor.

morphine, pearl Harbor

Ann Neuser Lederer
12/10/2010

They do not scream. They keep their hands steady as they shoot the shots.
They run from one to the next, on their rounds without walls.
The troops of well trained girls patrol the troops, their wards.

And they make them to inhale their brew
of Friar's Balsam, tincture of tree resin:
Pines and cooling mountain breezes in the steaming, smoke filled chaos.
Pliable amber beads, shrines for prehistoric bees,
crumbs for tuneful fiddles lull like opium beds
on the dark, explosive rocks

And though they run around, the nurses are careful.

They inscribe the letter M on the foreheads of those they have dosed,
They make their gentle mark on foreheads doomed or wounded,
under dust and thunder.

About the poet: Ann Neuser Lederer was born in Ohio and has also lived and worked in Pennsylvania, Michigan and Kentucky. Her poems and creative nonfiction can be found in journals such as Brevity, Diagram *and* Hospital Drive, *in anthologies such as* A Call to Nursing *(2009) and* The Country Doctor Revisited *(2010) and in her chapbooks* Approaching Freeze, The Undifferentiated *and* Weaning the Babies. *She has earned degrees in anthropology and in nursing and is currently employed as an RN in her fourth university hospital in as many states. For more of her writing, see* sites.google.com/site/anneneuserlederer/

About the poem: This poem was inspired by a passage in The Writer's Almanac *describing a scene from the attack on Pearl Harbor. "The nurses ran around, administering morphine, and to prevent overdoses, they wrote the letter M on each treated man's forehead."*

food

Joanne Wilkinson
12/17/2010

I have a stress test nearly every year. I do this because my mother dropped dead of a heart attack when she was thirty-six, and now I am thirty-five.

They stick EKG leads on me, and for weeks I have blotchy red circles on my skin where it's reacted to the adhesive. I run on the treadmill. Sometimes the cardiologist scans my heart and arteries with ultrasound; other times, he injects me with a radioactive marker. Sometimes he looks at me as though I'm wasting his time. Sometimes he frowns and looks concerned when he hears about my family history.

I always pass the test.

Why did my mother have a heart attack? I don't have satisfying answers for this. Was her cholesterol high? I don't know. They didn't check young women's cholesterol in the 1970s; they just gave them Valium for the tightness in their chests and told them not to worry. Was it because she had uncontrolled hypertension? Because she didn't exercise? Because she was doomed?

Am I doomed?

Last night I had dinner at an extravagant restaurant in New Orleans.

I'd never been to New Orleans before, and part of me was delighted by the experience: holding hands with my husband as we walked through the French Quarter on our first weekend away together in almost a year; sitting back in the restaurant and letting a tuxedoed waiter fuss over me with a breadcrumb scraper.

But the other part of me cut every morsel of steak and looked at it as an evil invader cloaked in creamy, atherosclerotic sauce. The other part of me woke up this morning and raced to the hotel's gym, certain that the vague discomfort in my stomach as I bobbed on the StairMaster was due not to overeating but to incipient angina. The other part of me has coronaries on the brain.

I feel a lot of different things about food. Just before coming to New Orleans, I was struck by a bout of rotavirus, kneeling on the bathroom floor for hours, collapsing on my futon tachycardic and light-headed. For three full days I lived on nothing but Gatorade; when we finally arrived in New Orleans, we ordered spinach tortellini from room service. As the first fragrant bite permeated the mucus membranes of my mouth, I felt I'd come back to life.

On the other hand, my pants were fetchingly baggy during those few days that I was ill. Once, I had an acute gallbladder attack. For two weeks I could eat nothing but crackers, and I lost fourteen pounds. Sometimes I think if I could have lasted just a little longer before surgery, I could have made it to twenty.

I love food. In college, I became an athlete. I still row and lift weights most days. Every morning, I leave the gym feeling cleansed, with that pleasantly wobbly feeling in my legs, the good kind of ache. When dinnertime rolls around, I love the sensory experience of a bowl of chili, pasta and vegetables, grilled chicken. My husband is a good cook, and I let him feed me. When I was growing up with my father, we ate out most nights and ordered pizza the rest. He was not the kind of person who relished the act of cooking and eating a meal. Food was fuel, nothing more. Now, I taste not only rosemary and garlic but also the balm of my husband's love and good will warming me, radiating outward from my stomach.

On the other hand, I'm terrible about feeding myself. For years, I felt that the whole idea of sitting down to eat was self-indulgent, not something I deserved. A cookie grabbed on the run between patients was what I should get, not a meal. I often forget to pack lunch, forget to eat lunch or dinner when I'm working. I look up from my desk at odd times of the day, starved, and realize the cafeteria is closed and that I'll have to buy a granola bar from the vending machine.

Sometimes I look at every piece of food I put in my mouth and think, "Well, this is it—this is the one that will put me over the edge." When I die, they'll say, "It was that last crème brûlée in New Orleans. What was she thinking?"

Sometimes, even though I love food, I wish that I could subsist on fat-free protein shakes three times a day. No more real food, no more decisions. No more living.

And other times, because I am home with a sore throat and feeling sorry for myself and haven't had a mommy to take care of me since practically forever, I ask my husband to make macaroni and cheese for me, and he does, and I eat it and feel loved.

I don't know the answer. I don't know if the slow accumulation of eating out and desserts over the years will kill me, or if so, when. I don't know if I'm actually allowed to be nourished, to eat good food, to let my husband take care of me in a way I barely remember. I don't know if I will live to be ninety eating Whitman's chocolates, like my grandmother. These thoughts are always with me, and sometimes I wish I could lay them down.

This morning, after the gym, I walked down to the riverfront with my husband and ordered beignets. We were in New Orleans, so I had some. They were delicious.

We sat in a little corner breakfast shop, on vacation together, the sun warming our backs. We talked about our lives, our plans, about how nice vacation is. The breeze blew in from the water and lifted my hair. I licked my finger to pick up the last bit of powdered sugar from my plate.

Then we walked away, into the day.

About the author: *Joanne Wilkinson is an assistant professor of family medicine at the Boston University School of Medicine. Her short stories and essays have been published in* Journal of Family Practice, Family Medicine, Medicine & Health Rhode Island *and* Medical Economics. *She has won several awards for creative writing and in 2008 was awarded the Mid-Career Faculty Achievement Award by the Family Medicine Education Consortium. She lives in the Boston area with her family.*

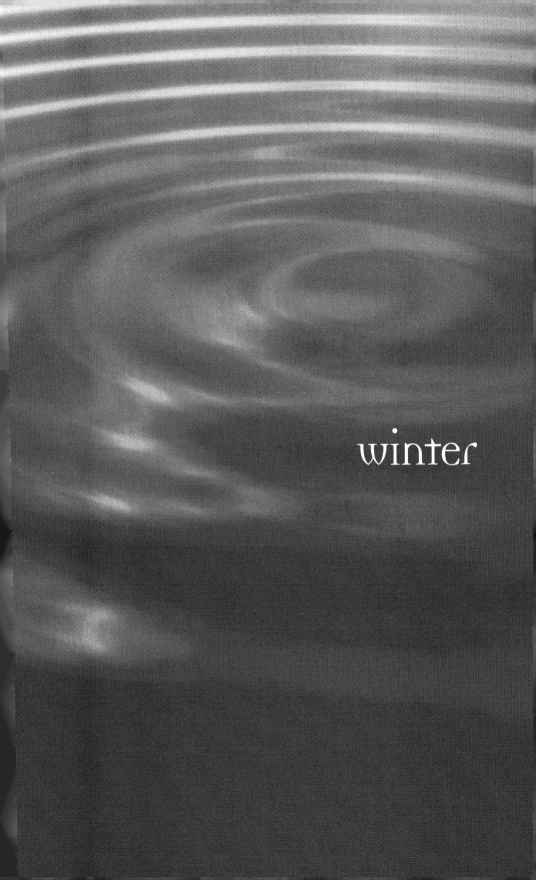

winter

Things That Matter

Paul Gross
12/24/2010

For me, the best part of being a doctor, and the biggest privilege, is getting to talk with people about things that matter.

"You look sad today," I say to a patient I'm seeing for the first time—a thirty-eight-year-old woman with a headache. In response, her lower lip starts to tremble, and she wipes an eye.

As I reach for the box of tissues and hand it to her, I know that whatever has caused her tears will be more important than her presenting symptom.

A forty-five-year-old man comes in wanting help sustaining erections. When I ask for a few details, it turns out he's having sex every single day of the week, and he's finding it a challenge to maintain an erection for twenty to thirty minutes. When he misses a day, he has sex twice the next day "to catch up." He has relations with his wife and also with a girlfriend who lives out of town, where he often travels on business.

Should I laugh? Let my eyes pop out of my head? Wag a finger?

Because I cherish the talking and like to think that I'm skilled at it, it's all the more comical when I end up with egg on my face:

In the course of a visit, I learn that a nineteen-year-old is having sexual relations with her steady male partner.

"Are you using birth control?" I ask

"No."

"Do you want to become pregnant?" I ask. "Are you ready to become a parent?"

"I'm not sure," she answers.

In violation of my own rule about never lecturing patients, I proceed to give a lecture. Or maybe it's two lectures—about the likelihood of pregnancy, about the impact of an unplanned child on her life. *Blah-blah-blah.*

She listens politely.

Later in the conversation, I discover that her boyfriend uses condoms. *Always*. And that *his* using condoms, in her mind, doesn't equate with *her* using birth control.

Oh, lord, I not only missed the boat, I also got on the wrong bus....

Some time ago, we launched *Pulse* with the idea of creating a safe space where all of us—patients, clinicians, caregivers and students—could talk about things that matter. About events that have marked us. About words that have healed or wounded us. About our triumphs and pratfalls.

And now, some time later, here we are—a little older and wiser, and still talking about things that matter.

As the year draws to a close, I'd like to thank you for your readership. I hope that the arrival of *Pulse* each Friday has mattered to you. Rest assured that your appreciation has mattered deeply to us.

As the year draws to a close, we at *Pulse* thank you for taking this journey with us—and for sharing and reading stories and poems that make a difference.

Warmly,

Paul Gross MD
Editor-in-Chief

as edited by...

Diane Guernsey
Executive Editor

The Ancients Had It Right

Stanley H. Schuman
12/31/2010

In Aramaic scripture,* and Aboriginal Dreamtime.
How else could animal life begin
Except by Divine Breath, oxygen-enriched?
How ingenious! Only two atoms: O2,
Ideal for hemoglobin, mitochondria,
Neurotransmitters, ideal for fight or flight, for vocalizing,
For clever humans to shape tools, split atoms,
Compose opera, sow seeds, harvest grain.

Consider my distress, in my just-opened pediatric office.
Stumped by Angela, a three-year-old
So panicked by my white coat, no way to examine her.

Screaming, clutching Mother, she knew and I knew
This wasn't university-hospital, with back-up nurses.
Instead, it was one-on-one,
Advantage Angela.

Desperate, I felt for a stray balloon in my
Pants pocket (from my own child's birthday).
Putting it to my lips, I strained to inflate the stubborn thing.
Instantly, Angela's tear-reddened eyes opened wide.
The more I flushed and puffed, clown-like,
The more she giggled, finally bursting into laughter,
Sans fear, forgetting pain.
My breath, a yellow balloon, a child's laughter...
Three gifts from the gods!

Douglas-Klotz, N.: Prayers of the Cosmos, 1990 Harper, San Francisco, CA.

About the poet: *Stan Schuman began as a pediatrician before turning to epidemiology. He is now professor emeritus in the family medicine department at Medical University of South Carolina. He helped to pioneer agromedicine—environmental medicine as applied to toxic exposures in farming-related fields. His several books include* Rainbows in Washtubs: Diagnostic Mysteries in Agromedicine

(Haworth Medical Press, 2006). "Writing poems has given me a welcome break from left-brain epidemiologic investigation and allowed me to engage in relaxed, right-brain play with colors and emotions....After fifty years spent between the University of Michigan and MUSC, I find the peace of a campus town and family (my wife of fifty-eight years, eight children and eighteen grandchildren) conducive to poems, in my head and on paper."

About the poem: "This poem captures two memories for me: my anxious first day in solo pediatric practice in suburban St. Louis, 1954, and my enchantment with the Aborigines' faith in the awesome power of nature in a person's waking and dreaming."

indexes

index by author

index by title, with summaries

Poems (first lines included)

index by Healthcare role

Nurses

Patients

Physician Assistants

Residents

Index by subject/theme

Communication

Complementary therapies

Confidentiality

Death and dying

Dementia

Disability

Doctor as patient

Doctor-patient relationship

Domestic violence

Geriatrics

Health policy

HIV

Homelessness

Humor

Medical errors

Medical training

Memorable patients

Mental health

Personal remembrance

Psychotherapy

Public health

Role modeling

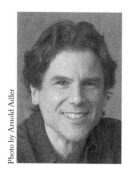

Photo by Arnold Adler

Paul Gross is founding editor of *Pulse—voices from the heart of medicine*. A family physician in the Bronx, he is on the faculty at Montefiore's Residency Program in Social Medicine and at Albert Einstein College of Medicine. He writes about the personal side of medicine, teaches reflective writing to residents and medical students, and conducts writing workshops for health professionals, students and patients.

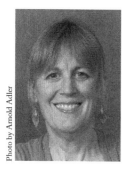

Photo by Arnold Adler

Diane Guernsey is executive editor of *Pulse—voices from the heart of medicine*. A former senior editor and longtime contributor at *Town & Country Magazine*, she now writes about health, medicine and related topics for *Consumer Reports* and other publications. Diane's career extends to other fields as well. She is a classical pianist, teaching piano and coaching singers at Manhattanville College in Purchase, NY, and she is also a licensed psychoanalyst.

Made in the USA
Charleston, SC
24 September 2012